KU-201-765

# CANCER:

# 50 ESSENTIAL THINGS TO DO

## THIRD EDITION

## GREG ANDERSON

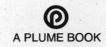

A PLUME BOOK

PLUME
Published by the Penguin Group
Penguin Group (USA) Inc., 375 Hudson Street, New York, New York 10014, U.S.A.
Penguin Group (Canada), 90 Eglinton Avenue East, Suite 700, Toronto, Ontario, Canada M4P 2Y3 (a division of Pearson Penguin Canada Inc.)
Penguin Books Ltd., 80 Strand, London WC2R 0RL, England
Penguin Ireland, 25 St. Stephen's Green, Dublin 2, Ireland (a division of Penguin Books Ltd.)
Penguin Group (Australia), 250 Camberwell Road, Camberwell, Victoria 3124, Australia (a division of Pearson Australia Group Pty. Ltd.)
Penguin Books India Pvt. Ltd., 11 Community Centre, Panchsheel Park, New Delhi – 110 017, India
Penguin Group (NZ), 67 Apollo Drive, Rosedale, North Shore 0632, New Zealand (a division of Pearson New Zealand Ltd)
Penguin Books (South Africa) (Pty.) Ltd., 24 Sturdee Avenue, Rosebank, Johannesburg 2196, South Africa

Penguin Books Ltd., Registered Offices: 80 Strand, London WC2R 0RL, England

First published by Plume, a member of Penguin Group (USA) Inc. An earlier edition of this book was published by Plume under the title *50 Essential Things to Do When the Doctor Says It's Cancer.*

First Printing, August 1999
Third Edition, March 2009
10   9   8   7   6   5   4   3

Copyright © Greg Anderson, 1999, 2009
All rights reserved

 REGISTERED TRADEMARK—MARCA REGISTRADA

LIBRARY OF CONGRESS CATALOGING-IN-PUBLICATION DATA

Anderson, Greg.
  Cancer: 50 essential things to do / Greg Anderson.
    p. cm.
  "Revised edition of 50 Essential things to do when the doctor says it's cancer."
  ISBN 978-0-452-29010-5
  1. Cancer—Popular works. I. Anderson, Greg. 50 things to do when the doctor says it's cancer. II. Title.
  RC263.A617 1999
  616.99'44—dc21                98-53091

Printed in the United States of America
Set in Caslon 540 Roman
Designed by Leonard Telesca

Without limiting the rights under copyright reserved above, no part of this publication may be reproduced, stored in, or introduced into a retrieval system, or transmitted, in any form, or by any means (electronic, mechanical, photocopying, recording, or otherwise), without the prior written permission of both the copyright owner and the above publisher of this book.

PUBLISHER'S NOTE
The scanning, uploading, and distribution of this book via the Internet or via any other means without the permission of the publisher is illegal and punishable by law. Please purchase only authorized electronic editions, and do not participate in or encourage electronic piracy of copyrighted materials. Your support of the author's rights is appreciated.

BOOKS ARE AVAILABLE AT QUANTITY DISCOUNTS WHEN USED TO PROMOTE PRODUCTS OR SERVICES. FOR INFORMATION PLEASE WRITE TO PREMIUM MARKETING DIVISION, PENGUIN GROUP (USA) INC., 375 HUDSON STREET, NEW YORK, NEW YORK 10014.

A PLUME BOOK

# CANCER: 50 ESSENTIAL THINGS TO DO

GREG ANDERSON is the founder of the Cancer Recovery Foundation International group of charities, a global affiliation of national organizations whose mission is to help all people prevent and survive cancer.

The Cancer Recovery Foundation focuses on integrated cancer care programs, improving the lives of all people touched by cancer. It funds no clinical research or medical treatments. The foundation has established affiliates in Australia, Canada, France, Germany, the United Kingdom, and the United States.

Greg Anderson was diagnosed with stage IV lung cancer in 1984. His surgeon gave him just thirty days to live. Refusing to accept the hopelessness of this prognosis, he went searching for people who had lived even though their doctors had told them they were "terminal." His findings from interviews with over 16,000 cancer survivors form the strategies and action points for what has become an international cancer recovery movement.

Anderson is widely recognized as one of the world's leading wellness authorities. He is the author of ten books, including the inspirational classic *The Cancer Conqueror* and *Cancer and the Lord's Prayer*.

*This book is dedicated to my wife, Linda.*
*Your unconditional loving sustains me.*

# CONTENTS

# FOREWORD

For over thirty-five years, I have been working with an approach to cancer that includes the physical, mental, and spiritual. I have treated thousands of patients with a relatively high rate of recovery, even from so-called "terminal" illness. I have learned a great deal about healing, and I have met some remarkable patients. Greg Anderson is one of them.

This book, *Cancer: 50 Essential Things to Do*, is a testimony to patients taking charge and choosing a stance of hope toward a diagnosis of cancer. Many of you who read this book are undoubtedly in a very difficult situation. Do not despair. Keep your hope alive. Learn from the experience of someone who was given a thirty-days-to-live prognosis. The author has been there. He knows what it's like to deal with the despair of cancer. He also knows what it takes to get well again.

While the road ahead may be difficult, I want you to know that it can be the most rewarding journey you will ever take. Even though the path through cancer requires work and discipline, it is also filled with discoveries that will excite and motivate you. Keep your focus on those joys.

Begin your journey now. Here, in this book, are the keys that can open the door for your return to good health. Take charge. Live this moment. Forgive. Love. You'll then know the power of hope . . . and you will be on the path to getting well again.

> —O. Carl Simonton, M.D.
> Founder, Simonton Cancer Center
> Pacific Palisades, California

# ACKNOWLEDGMENTS

A heartfelt thank-you to all the friends and colleagues of Cancer Recovery Foundation. I treasure you.

To all who so generously gave their time, talents and creativity to this project, please accept my sincere appreciation.

And to all who search these pages for the answers to wellness, my encouragement and love.

# INTRODUCTION

This revised and updated edition of *Cancer: 50 Essential Things to Do* is written for those people who want to survive the experience of cancer and are willing to participate actively in the recovery process. My goal is twofold: to help you consider the major issues following a cancer diagnosis, and to encourage you to implement a comprehensive, integrated cancer recovery plan of your own design that has your highest confidence level.

I ask you to start with the end in mind. Beyond treatment of illness, I will help you create wellness. The creation of well-being—physically, emotionally and spiritually—is exactly what conquers cancer.

This book is action-oriented, designed to help you put in motion a program that will maximize your opportunity for a complete recovery while maintaining a high quality of life. This is not a book to be read and then put away, never to be referred to again. Instead, think of using this as your resource guide for the next two years—a reasonable time for recovery. Return to it again and again to get "unstuck" in your cancer journey.

This book has a meaningful message for every person touched by cancer. The strategies are tailor-made for the person with a recent cancer diagnosis. If you have recently been told, "It's cancer," you'll find here the information you need to gain control over your fears, analyze your diagnosis, and put in place the most effective integrated cancer care program possible.

For the newly diagnosed, I recommend following the "50 Essential Things" in order. There is a certain logical progression in their sequence. Following this pattern will prove invaluable and will ensure that you are making the wisest decisions possible.

I also wrote this book for the person who has been diagnosed with a recurrence of cancer. Recurrence is a very, very frightening event, a time of reevaluation medically, emotionally, and spiritually. I encourage you to make the "50 Essential Things" the very heart of your entire analysis. Thoughtfully follow the steps. Use this book as your primary guide.

Know this: a recurrence does not equate with certain death. What you do does make a difference! See the "50 Essential Things" as mandatory points of action. Then you'll know you're doing everything possible to get well again.

## The Wellness and Recovery Journal

Before you begin reading, secure a notebook and a pencil, or create a new folder on your laptop. I want you to create a Wellness and Recovery Journal. I started mine with a single sheet of my daughter's notebook paper and an old three-ring binder. Nothing elaborate is required.

As you read, questions and insights will come to mind. Write them down. You'll find yourself clipping newspaper and magazine articles about cancer. Put them in your notebook. This is going to become your primary source book, a reference manual for your personal and individualized cancer recovery program. Now, over twenty-four years after I was told I would die, my journal contains a wealth of insights important to me. I still add information.

My journal also serves as an excellent log that records my cancer recovery journey.

Do the same. You need the clarity the Wellness and Recovery Journal delivers. Even though a road map to recovery is contained in this book, each person must ultimately chart his or her own course. Use your Wellness and Recovery Journal to record your unique personal insights.

Especially record your questions. Then ask. Ask your doctor, your medical technicians, and other survivors. Nothing is to be assumed. Ask about medical terms that you don't understand. Ask about reasons for tests. Ask about the results of those tests. Ask for success stories. Ask. Ask. Ask. Asking questions gives you significant power. Do not be intimidated by medical personnel or the process. You are the one in charge. Ask! Then record the responses. Come back to them again and again.

Through it all, there is good reason to be filled with hope, provided you take an active part in the recovery process. Understand this recurring theme: *you must not simply treat illness, you must also create wellness.*

Let's get started now.

Hershey, Pennsylvania
January 2009

# AUTHOR'S NOTE

The ideas in this book are meant to supplement the care and guidance of competent medical professionals. At no time does the author suggest that these steps take the place of conventional medical treatment. Do not attempt a self-diagnosis. Do not embark upon self-treatment of a serious illness without professional help. There are a growing number of informed doctors who will work with their clients to integrate body, mind, and spirit. Find one. Form a healing partnership.

The characters in this book are composites of real people. They are not intended to portray specific individuals.

# ESSENTIAL
# UNDERSTANDING

# What's
# Happening

## Integrated Cancer Care

For nearly a quarter-century following a terminal lung cancer diagnosis, my reason for being has been to offer healing and support to people experiencing cancer. With my wife, Linda, I extend that same offer to the loved ones who support cancer patients. I assume you, the reader, are in one of those categories.

Our approach has always been "holisitic." This means we recognize the central importance of integrating body, mind, and spirit—the physical, emotional, and spiritual components of health and well-being.

From interviews with over 16,000 cancer survivors, I have come to understand that health is much more than not being sick. The corollary: I have come to understand that cancer is much, much more than cells gone awry.

Our work has led to a very important conclusion: surviving cancer is not simply about treating illness. It is primarily about creating wellness—holistic well-being.

Allow me to repeat for emphasis: if you believe there is value in learning from the experience of cancer survivors, you must not only treat illness, you must also create wellness.

All that I am suggesting is in addition to, not in place of, conventional medical care. That's what the term "integrated cancer care" stands for. Evidence abounds that integrating complementary and even alternative approaches into a conventional bio-medical cancer treatment program is very likely to result in better outcomes, reduced side effects, a greater sense of control, and a much improved quality of life.

Along with a world-class team of associates at the Cancer Recovery Foundation, I have extensively investigated "what went right" for cancer survivors. Today I wish to emphatically state that orthodox medical treatment alone does not maximize one's opportunity for cancer survival. It's not enough.

While the Cancer Recovery Foundation certainly supports each individual's choices and decisions in treatment, be they strictly conventional, complementary, or alternative, we have become much more assertive in urging the integrated approach. You will see that emphasis throughout this book. The work takes three forms:

- Education. Helping you understand the array of influences that may cause cancer, the spectrum of treatment options, and what you can do to help yourself.
- Empowerment. Helping and supporting you in actually implementing these strategies in your cancer recovery journey, making them a new way of life.
- Encouragement. Supporting you by offering inspiration and hope that, no matter how difficult, you can survive and even thrive through cancer.

Those are very big promises. The holistic approach delivers.

The purpose of this book is to fully explain and explore the implications of this holistic strategy. It is also to help you apply these ideas in simple, understandable steps. These ideas offer you a plan to get well and stay well for the remainder of your life however long or short that time may be.

The end result is a unique body-mind-spirit approach to health and healing. Implementing this strategy improves the ability to deal with the diagnosis, make informed choices about treatments, and mobilize all the resources available to you in the healing process.

In the end, the integrated cancer care strategy helps turn the crisis of cancer into a unique opportunity to live far more happily and healthfully than ever before.

## THE HOLISTIC MODEL

In the early years of our work, I looked to the cellular biology of cancer as the starting point. That was a mistake. Integrated cancer care is built on a foundation that extends well beyond the modern biomedical model of what's wrong.

Today, our starting point is to view each person's state of health as a result of the many interactive components of body, mind, and spirit. Cell biology may be a component, but it is more often the result, the end game, of a host of other lifestyle choices. These include nutrition, exercise, attitude, social support, and especially spirituality. I've also expanded my definition of health to evaluate the environment in which we live as well as the manner in which we internally process all these factors.

There is currently a growing belief that genetics explains cancer and is the basis of the promise of a cure. Truth is, genetics has so far been a huge disappointment. Even the preeminent leaders in the field concede the massive influence of lifestyle on disease. In fact, lifestyle choices seem to reverse or control the triggering of genetic predispositions to illness. An obvious example: if you smoke cigarettes, gene therapy will not help you prevent or recover from lung cancer.

So today, our starting point is your state of health. Question #1: How is it?

If you will step back and observe, you will see many complex influences working around you and through you. Your health and well-being are functions of these factors. More than just physical well-being, there are also the issues of emotional and spiritual wellness.

One way to assess your state of holistic well-being is to ask yourself a series of questions. These may include:

Physical well-being:

Do I truly practice high nutritional intelligence?
Do I exercise each day?
Do I seek health guidance from competent health guides?

Attitudinal well-being:

Do I balance time for myself with time for others?
Do I allow time for play or am I a workaholic?
Do I ask others for help or must I always go it alone?

Emotional well-being:

Do I feel free to express my feelings or do I keep a stiff upper lip?
Do I possess an awareness of my dominant emotional style?
Do I understand how to choose and manage my emotions?

Social well-being:

Do I feel a close connection with others?
Do I both give and receive attention?
Do I have someone with whom I can share everything?

Spiritual well-being:

Do I have a sense there is "more"—a divine part to life?
Do I have an intimate connection with the divine?
Do I know what to do to establish and strengthen my spiritual connection?

Grade yourself on each of these questions. What is your grade point average?

While certainly not exhaustive, this more complete picture of one's state of health is central to an understanding of how to get well again and stay well. The result is the ability to mobilize the whole person—body, mind, and spirit—not only for recovery from illness, but also to maximize your well-being.

This understanding is at odds with medical orthodoxy. This model takes you well beyond cell biology and is in stark contrast to the conventional medical approach that is the norm in Western medicine today. The biomedical understanding of health focuses exclusively on the physical dimensions of well-being and envisions the body as a machine. Disease is considered a malfunction of the machine.

According to this model, illness is a specific failure that can be remedied by correcting that failure. With cancer, this worldview very logically leads to mechanical fixes that predominantly rely on surgery, radiation therapy, chemotherapy, and hormonal therapy.

I have come to believe these treatments have a time and place in many individual cancer recovery programs. However, I have also come to understand that they are not to occupy the dominant place. Instead, after nearly a quarter-century of study, I now believe these treatments are temporary steps to allow the body itself the opportunity to alleviate the burden of cancer. Once the burden is lessened, the whole person can then go forward to create wellness.

I know this is a radical position. I also believe it is totally accurate and completely trustworthy. Reducing tumor burden and then doing all possible to nurture the body to heal itself is the rational alternative to a never-ending program of increasingly toxic, invasive, and experimental cancer treatments.

## A DIFFERENT KIND OF ILLNESS

I want you to understand that cancer is a complex and multi-dimensional process. It has a wide spectrum of causes and influences, including genetic, nutritional, stress-related, environmental, and even emotional. Some of these causes are direct, some indirect.

The physical symptoms resulting from these causes are the cellular component of cancer. At the cell level, think of cancer as the mutation of genes resulting in the irregular growth of abnormal cells. The operative words here are *irregular* and *abnormal.*

Healthy cells of the body grow in predictable patterns. As they wear out, they are replaced in an orderly manner by just the right number of new healthy cells.

Cancerous cells grow in uncontrolled and unpredictable patterns. Their growth serves no useful biological purpose. They often threaten the entire body. The cells themselves are mutant, changed in ways that limit their function.

You have this cellular condition in your body. It is one of more than one hundred types of cancers, each having its own site and distinguishing characteristics.

A second dimension of cancer is an inefficient immune system. Your understanding of this second point is of vital importance; it is critical in your decision to do all you can to help yourself get well. Your immune system is the first and most powerful defense your body has against cancer. For years you have periodically produced mutant cells that were potentially cancerous. In most cases, the immune system was there to "clean up" the problems. Now your immune system has ceased doing so in an efficient enough manner to ensure your health.

I believe rebuilding your immune function is absolutely central to your getting well and staying well. This book will give you specific steps to help you respond with maximum intelligence to this diagnosis and help you rebuild your self-healing functions. The basic action points are:

1. Examine. Step back from the day-to-day pressures of life to evaluate your current situation in its entirety.
2. Discover. Assess both current life issues that must be changed as well as future needs that must be met.
3. Plan. Create a plan to restore health and total well-being.
4. Implement. Work in partnership with health advisors who have your confidence. Begin a self-care plan to create whole-person well-being.
5. Review. Conduct quarterly reviews of your progress, making adjustments as necessary.

Right now, I ask you to open your Wellness and Recovery Journal. Take five pages and put one of the above action points at the top of each page. Then number 1 through 10 below each action point.

Taken together, these action points will play the central role in mobilizing all your healing options, both external and internal. You will then live well for as long as you live. Living well . . . that is powerful healing in and of itself.

I have come to understand and experience this to be the body-mind-spirit connection at work. It is real. It is powerful. When used in conjunction with prudent medical care, you can be assured you have created the optimum environment for healing. Your medical team will do all it can to fix the malfunctioning machine. Your task is to do all you can to enhance your self-healing capacity.

Enhancing your self-healing capacity is accomplished through your own choices—your physical, emotional, and spiritual lifestyle. In a very real sense, I am asking you to make a commitment to "lifestyle therapy," initiating and implementing a holistic whole-person recovery effort.

Abundant authoritative, scientifically validated evidence exists that the immune system is profoundly influenced by lifestyle choices. Few people would argue that tobacco use, improper diet, and lack of exercise are obvious deterrents to maximum health. So is mismanaged toxic stress, which fills the body with adrenaline and cortisone derivatives, both known to inhibit immune function.

Something as basic as your emotional response to the communication of a cancer diagnosis is a factor. The message, "It's cancer," is received with pervasive fear by most people. That fear can paralyze the recipient emotionally and psychologically at a time when intelligent action is required. And a spiritually toxic outlook after a cancer diagnosis can make a difficult situation a living hell. These responses have a negative physiological impact on immune function.

Ideally, even before putting your medical team in place, your concentrated efforts will be directed toward the mental, emotional, and spiritual practices that optimize your chances of recovery. Fail to do so at your own peril. Retaining a medical team without doing all you can to help yourself is like attempting to walk with one stilt. It's possible but the results are frequently disappointing.

The comprehensive, integrated holistic cancer care emphasis of this book, and the implementation of the strategies that flow from this approach, should not cast dispersions on the validity of truly scientific medicine. I do not encourage you to go back to the use of folk medicine, though I do have the utmost respect for the old-fashioned family doctor who would ask, listen, show compassion, and treat the whole person.

But there is a one glaring problem with so-called science-based medicine: it's not scientific enough. Again and again, science says one thing today and the complete opposite tomorrow. As you will read, I severely question much of the widespread use of chemotherapy for this very reason. Scientifically valid evidence supporting the holistic approach does exist. The trouble is, we cannot yet measure the obviously positive outcomes to our complete scientific satisfaction. And because the effects cannot be, or have not been, measured in large-scale randomized clinical trials, the evidence tends to be dismissed. Too bad.

Two pioneers in integrated cancer care need to be recognized. O. Carl Simonton, M.D., is the father of modern psychosocial oncology. For over thirty years, his work has yielded consistent evidence that mind-body techniques such as relaxation, self-hypnosis, and guided imagery significantly reduce stress and anxiety in cancer patients and contribute to recovery.

In Canada, Alastair Cunningham, Ph.D., traced substantial improvements in quality of life for those cancer patients who adopted the holistic strategy. His work also confirms the validity of the growing body of evidence that psycho-spiritual self-help not only prolongs life but is also correlated with unexpected remissions in thousands of cases of cancer.

I am keenly aware that evidence does not equate with proof. But understand this: lack of evidence is not equal to disproof. As we shall later discuss, many widely accepted orthodox cancer treatment protocols are based on less-than-complete science.

Modern medicine will become truly scientific only when patients and their medical teams learn to manage the natural forces of body, mind, and spirit within the context of a program for total well-being.

If you have cancer today, you can't wait for years of clinical research to prove these points. So don't wait. Becoming proactive in creating your own wellness will not only influence your quality of life, but it will also influence your quantity of life. This book will provide you with the most up-to-date knowledge available. Integrate these principles with the best medicine has to offer. Therein lies optimum success.

Cancer is indeed a different kind of illness that demands a different kind of response. Recovery demands your total participation. For cancer patients determined to conquer this illness, that is very good news indeed.

## No Such Thing as Hopeless

You may have been told, "Get your affairs in order," or "You have just a short time left," or a favorite of the medical community, "Your illness is terminal." Don't believe it. Refuse to give in to that despair. Only God knows how long a person has to live.

In 1984, I was given a thirty-days-to-live prognosis. It was lung cancer. I'd previously had one lung removed. Now, four months later, the cancer was back. This time it was in my ribs and lymph system. The surgeon put his hand on my shoulder and said, "Greg, the tiger is out of the cage. Your cancer has come roaring back. I would give you about thirty days to live."

Part of the reason that surgeon was mistaken is that no health-care provider can predict a person's response to illness. After several days of believing I would die, I made a profound decision. I decided to live.

Please understand clearly what I am saying. By deciding to live I made a decision to do all I could to triumph over the cancer. I determined to live each day I was given to the very best of my ability. I chose not to focus on the despair communicated in the surgeon's words. I would instead adopt a stance of hopefulness. These decisions dramatically changed my experience of illness. They resulted not only in better days but many more days as well. I believe such a decision by you may result in a similar outcome.

This message has its vocal critics. It's controversial. More than once, esteemed members of the health-care community have publicly accused me of spreading false hope. My answer is simple and direct. I believe there is no such thing as false hope. There is only reasonable hope. Reasonable hope is a medicine worthy of consumption in large doses.

What is clearly false is a doctor's pronouncement that sets a limit on the amount of time a patient may have left to live. That's "false hopelessness." It is false because no human being knows how long anyone has left to live. To prognosticate in such a manner is not only unprofessional, it is unethical.

My response to the surgeon was strong. I said, "Thank you, doctor. You've given me thirty days to live. Wow! That's wonderful because God only gives me one day at a time!" Healers instill hope. They do not schedule death.

There is no such thing as hopeless. Decide to live—today! Embrace hope deep within your spirit. It heals. It is a decision that always leads to greater quality in our days. I also believe it leads to a greater quantity of our days.

I deeply empathize with you and your health crisis. I have been there. I have been torn by the same emotions that now rip at you. I can identify with your fear and uncertainty. It is the most frightening time of your life.

Two paths are before you. One is marked by the road signs of passivity and despair; the other by the guideposts of engagement and hope. You have a choice. Please, choose hope.

If you have been told that your time is limited, believe that life can still be a fulfilling adventure. Choose to live life to the very fullest. Focus on the possibilities, not the problem. Affirm that each day is a good and perfect gift in spite of the circumstances of illness. Keep your thoughts on hope and healing. In that intentional choice are the seeds of your cancer recovery. Water those seeds, not the weeds.

Without question you can improve your potential for survival. What you do makes a significant difference. Believe it: there is no such thing as a hopeless situation.

# A
# ROAD
# MAP TO
# RECOVERY

## LEARNING FROM THE TRUE EXPERTS

After my surgeon told me I had thirty days to live, I was stunned. One moment I was in tears, the next I was enraged. I thought it was all a mistake, convinced my tests had been confused with another patient's. I was filled with fear and self-pity. One afternoon I yelled out loud, "Oh God, what can I do?"

That question was answered. No, God did not part the clouds and speak; I remain a committed skeptic regarding such claims. But figuratively, the clouds were parted and God did speak. It was nonverbal communication, a distinct impression that my task was to search for survivors. I became aware, vitally aware—a knowing—that I was to seek people who were "supposed" to die but had lived. And once I found them, I was to learn from their experience.

Over the years, I have interviewed and received surveys from over 16,000 survivors of "terminal" illness. These are the people who have been told the equivalent of "Get your affairs in order.

You are about to die." They are the brave patients who, at one time, had no hope—the people the medical community wrote off. But these same people lived.

These inspiring individuals, who possess no more courage or ability than you or me, teach some very powerful lessons from which we would be well-served to learn. These ideas and practices have worked successfully for me and hundreds of thousands of other cancer patients. I am convinced these lessons and strategies can be pivotal in your life and your health.

After I conducted over 500 interviews, it became clear there were shared patterns to most of the individual outcomes. For example, the vast majority of survivors do not believe they recovered their health by chance or by being passive. The triumphant patients worked for their wellness, earning it on a daily basis. Neither do most cancer survivors credit their doctors alone, or even primarily, for their recovery. Instead, these exceptional patients focus on personally mobilizing body, mind, and spirit in their quest for high-level wellness.

Consistent patterns emerged from the survivor interviews. In 1988, I first summarized them and combined them into an eight-strategy program. In 2006, after thousands of additional interviews, I further refined them into six easily understood concepts that anyone could understand and put to use. Today, through Cancer Recovery Foundation International, over five million people have used these principles as a road map, a strategic plan to enhance their health and enrich their lives. I want the same for you.

## THE SIX STRATEGIES

Before we come to the "50 Essential Things," I'd like to give you an overview of the six basic approaches that cancer survivors have in common. Here is what emerged from the survivor interviews.

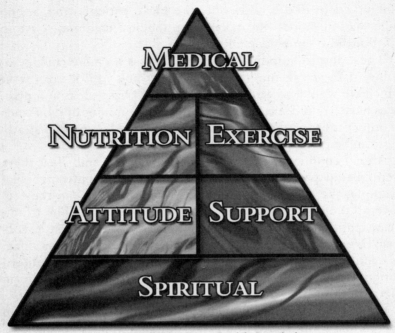

Copyright © 2007 Cancer Recovery Foundation International

## Strategy #1: Medical Treatment

Over 96 percent of cancer survivors start and complete at least one treatment program that is grounded in conventional medical care. Surgery, radiation therapy, chemotherapy, hormonal therapy, and immunotherapy—often in combination—are the treatments of choice. I was both surprised and encouraged by this.

Let me be very clear. Orthodox treatments have an important role in cancer survival. The overwhelming majority of cancer survivors do embrace conventional medical care. This is a very important message.

But there is a significant issue that has become much clearer since we first started our work some twenty-four years ago. It's the gross inconsistency in the medical treatment prescribed for similar diagnoses.

Take breast cancer as an example. Although several well-designed studies have clearly demonstrated that Breast Conserving Treatment (BCT) for stage I and II disease has the same success rate as mastectomy, the removal of the breast remains the predominant treatment.

There are marked regional differences, with women in larger cities more likely to receive BCT than those in rural areas. There is even a study showing double mastectomy, where both breasts are removed even when cancer exists in only one, is the fastest-growing breast cancer treatment.

All this despite the fact that the outcomes are statistically the same. This same treatment inconsistency is seen across virtually all cancers.

This is why patients everywhere must take matters into their own hands, demanding full knowledge and explanation of all treatment options. Thankfully, the amount of treatment information now available is significant. Demanding hard evidence regarding the effectiveness of suggested treatments is the key. So while 96 out of 100 surviving patients still opt for conventional treatments, their treatment decisions are more informed today than ever before. Do likewise.

Importantly, cancer survivors do not stop with conventional medical treatment. As you study the "50 Essential Things," you will see how survivors take charge of the management of their entire health and well-being. They choose doctors in whom they have confidence, often researching their educational background and clinical track record. Survivors consent only to treatment programs in which they have high confidence. Plus, survivors aggressively integrate complementary and alternative approaches with traditional medical care.

Survivors are active patients, involved with each decision, making certain they are fully informed and understand each component of their recovery program. Conventional medicine, yes. Patient control, even more. It is the prominent theme among cancer survivors.

## Strategy #2: Nutrition

Following medical care, dietary changes are the most common strategy adopted by the cancer survivors. The increasing importance of nutrition in cancer recovery has been one of the most significant shifts in the last decade. No longer is the old "Eat whatever you want" theory widely accepted.

Today, viewing "food as medicine" is the norm among cancer survivors. The most common nutritional shifts are toward diets that feature the following:

- Whole foods
- Foods low in fat, salt, and sugar
- An emphasis on fresh vegetables, fresh fruits, and whole grains
- Pure water

The single major dietary shift is consuming foods that are less processed. If it is boxed or bottled or canned or packaged, the food comes under immediate suspicion. These prepared foods tend to deliver calories with less nutrition than their fresh counterparts. In practice, cancer survivors spend most of their grocery shopping time in the produce section of their local market.

Nutritional supplements, while not taking the place of a whole food diet, are widely employed by cancer survivors. While there exists a lack of consensus in actual practice, survivors widely recognize the role of vitamin, mineral, and herbal supplements in the management of cancer. Thankfully, better science is producing evidence to support nutrition as a central element in cancer recovery.

One other observation on nutrition: cancer survivors eat with awareness. There is a marked increase in "nutritional IQ" among cancer patients, especially over the past ten years. Nutrition, not simply calories, has become the emerging battle cry of cancer patients in Western cultures. And survivors carry the attitude that a healthy diet is something they "get" to do, as opposed to something they "have" to do, to contribute to their survival. More spe-cifics on nutrition will be found later in this book.

## Strategy #3: Exercise

Survivors engage in some form of physical exercise virtually every day. The Cancer Recovery Foundation was the first orga-nization to document this trend over twenty years ago. It has ac-celerated. Today, the science is catching up with the survivors' practices and confirming the significant benefits of exercise.

Nearly nine out of ten cancer survivors I have interviewed and surveyed affirm the role of regular physical exercise in their own journey. I talked to bikers, swimmers, joggers, and walkers—lots of walkers. A brisk twenty-minute walk each day, with moderate strength training every other day, seems to be ideal. Do you know what? That's something all of us can do.

Most inspiring are the patients who started exercise programs even while confined to hospitals beds or wheelchairs. In spite of physical limits, these people exercised. If you seek to overcome cancer, phys-ical exercise needs to be an important part of your program.

## Strategy #4: Attitude

Survivors believe they will survive. Survivors embrace beliefs that generate attitudes and, in turn, create emotions that nurture healing. This is the mind-body connection. It is powerful.

Do beliefs and attitudes actually heal? Survivors see a direct link. They choose beliefs and attitudes about illness and wellness that empower. The most fundamental and empowering belief is that cancer does not mean death. It's sad but true that much of the world still considers cancer and death to be synonymous. Sur-vivors emphatically reject that belief.

This does not translate into denial, or some "be-positive-against-all-evidence" thinking. It's a warrior's attitude that sur-vivors demonstrate. There is a marked tough-mindedness in the cancer survivor community—"feistiness," as actress Suzanne Somers once described it. You see it everywhere.

Survivors face this truth: cancer may or may not mean death. This set of beliefs and attitudes results in emotions that carry vastly different outlooks from either the super-positive or hopelessly negative cancer patients. "Yes, I may die," said Chris Winters, a thirty-something California housewife. "But I am going to live to the fullest with cancer. I am not going to die of fear and hopelessness."

I want you to know that attitude is the essence of survivorship. These essential beliefs extend to medical treatments and potential side effects. Survivors envision their treatments as highly effective. They further believe side effects will be minimal and manageable. The "50 Essential Things" will help you understand and apply these attitudes of healing to your own integrated cancer care program.

You will not be surprised to learn that survivors believe they have the absolute central role in the recovery process. This belief and resulting attitude is at complete odds with millions of other cancer patients who defer virtually every question to their doctors. Not survivors.

It's surprising: survivors have interesting relationships with their medical team. They want the best of care and respect those health-care professionals who speak truth, patiently explaining what evidence supports their treatment recommendations and what outcomes can be expected. But if that information is not freely forthcoming, survivors can be exceptionally confrontational. Survivors check and recheck physician recommendations, often challenging tests, treatments, and prognoses. Many survivors change doctors in search of those who can be trusted and who meet their expectations.

## Strategy #5: Support

Relationships. Survivors invest time and emotional energy in relationships that nurture. They also invest less time and energy in relationships that are toxic. While this may seem to be a benign practice, it has some surprising holistic health implications.

Loving relationships with friends, relatives, lovers, spouses, children, coworkers, and employees—or the lack of those relationships—build us up or tear us down. Survivors become "relationship sensitive," examining, perhaps for the first time in their lives, how they relate to other people. It is quite common for survivors to put difficult relationships on hold, especially during any debilitating treatment phase. This does not mean survivors exile toxic people from their lives for all time. But it certainly signals reduced emotional and even spiritual investment in those relationships.

Cancer gives patients permission to examine a wide variety of life choices, especially their network of social support. Changes are often made. That is helpful because much of the work of getting well again takes place within the patient's social support network. The last thing a cancer patient needs is a critical person second-guessing every decision or predicting ultimate doom.

New and important research is now demonstrating the health benefits of supportive relationships. As much as I wish the research extended to the health benefits of cancer support groups, it currently does not show conclusive proof of benefits. But this much we know to be true of support: survivors have at least one person with whom they can share everything, literally everything, without fear of judgment. That is a powerful healing elixir.

## Strategy #6: Spiritual

Cancer survivors embrace a more spiritual perspective. They repeatedly speak of seeing life differently now compared to before their brush with death. This spiritual outlook stands in marked contrast to other cancer patients who obsess over a body that may be riddled with disease or endlessly mourn over dreams that are hopelessly derailed. Survivors surprise me in that they always seem to be able to grasp the high value of "now"—the simple and readily available life that is theirs even in spite of cancer. "I have today," said Doris, a fifty-year-old colon cancer patient. "That's a lot to be grateful for."

To label spirituality a "strategy" is inadequate. Survivors tend to undergo a spiritual transformation that is quite deep. For thousands of people, it becomes the central focus of their entire lives. In essence, they become new people.

This more spiritual perspective is not an issue of religion. Many survivors reject traditional religious practices. It's an old adage: just because you sit in a garage does not mean you will become a car. And just because you sit in a church does not mean you will become more spiritual. Clearly, no single doctrine or creed brings prepackaged answers.

Nor does this spirituality simply consist of bland platitudes. Instead, the transformation is typically seen as actively cultivating an inner peace, a serenity, a quiet confidence, a more grateful and joyful way of living. In a very real sense, survivors have come to let God work in and through them. Marianne Kegan, an ovarian cancer survivor, explained the essential nature of the spiritual walk. She said, "Now, when I walk into a room, I am there serving as God's representative." For millions of cancer survivors, this is the apex of the healing journey.

## IMPLEMENTATION INTELLIGENCE

Each of these six strategies is important and essential to cancer survival. However, they are not always equal. Timing is an issue. If the decision is made to consider and commence medical treatment, nearly all the emphasis tends to be placed on that area. Once in place, survivors let the doctors treat while they focus on nutrition, exercise, attitude, and the holistic aspects of getting well again.

Implementation of one principle typically follows another at the appropriate time. Few survivors make simultaneous wholesale changes. Those who do attempt to change too much too quickly often meet with temporary defeat and have to start again.

Many survivors note that solving a relationship issue may have been just as important in their recovery as medical treatment.

Adopting a healthy nutritional program and making a commitment to daily exercise may be on par with the contribution of radiation or chemotherapy.

It takes us back to where we started. We first review our state of health. That state is a result of the many interactive components of body, mind, and spirit. Yes, cell biology may be a component, but it is more often the result, the end game, of a host of other lifestyle choices.

Nearly all survivors agree it is the balance, the comprehensive integrated approach, that makes for survivorship. The survivors believe they have earned their return to health, aligning themselves with their own immense healing capacity. "Healing springs from within," said Randall Washington. "I simply had to work with God to release it."

Let's summarize to this point. The integration of these six key strategies represented by the cancer survival pyramid creates the framework for the cancer recovery process:

| | |
|---|---|
| Medical | Attitude |
| Nutrition | Support |
| Exercise | Spiritual |

The cancer survival pyramid is the context, the strategic plan, in which the "50 Essential Things" are implemented. The pyramid is your big picture, your road map. Consult it often.

# THE
# 50
# ESSENTIAL
# THINGS
# TO DO

# DESIGN
# YOUR
# INTEGRATED
# TREATMENT
# PROGRAM

Your number one priority following a cancer diagnosis is to put in place the best integrated cancer care program you can possibly design. This is much more than simply going to one doctor and saying, "Treat me."

The decisions you make regarding your cancer care and recovery program are some of the most important you will make in your entire life. Begin the journey through cancer by following this course of action, which has proven highly effective for hundreds of thousands of cancer survivors.

# #1

---

# STOP
# "AWFULIZING"

You've been told "It's cancer." I have deep compassion for you. I fully appreciate your feelings. I've been there, too.

First, you're in shock and filled with fear. The next moment you're angry but not quite certain at what or whom. Then comes the thoughts of, "How did this happen? Why me?" Even the guilt starts to creep in, "Did I bring this on myself?" Plus all the questions have started to rush through your mind: "Will I die?" "How long do I have?" "What will happen to my family?" And on and on and on. Your mind is overwhelmed at times.

Be calm. Try not to panic. I know that this is easier said than done. But be aware that panic will only inhibit rational and positive action.

Cancer is a serious illness, but it is not necessarily fatal. You do have the luxury of some time. Unlike a severed artery, cancer does not require you to do something this very instant. A hurried response, based in the emotions of fear and panic, is neither required nor preferred. In fact, a hurried response may be harmful. Don't take that as a license for inaction, however.

Stop and examine your frenzied thoughts for just a moment. It is at the beginning stages of this journey that clear decision-making will be most important. With these early decisions, you will ensure that your illness is properly treated. Panic acts only to your detriment.

Panic is a mental phenomenon, a response to our beliefs about cancer being frightful and overpowering. The process can accurately be labeled as "awfulizing." Isn't that an apt description? When we awfulize, we mentally take our current situation to its worst possible conclusion.

If we will objectively observe our emotions for just a moment, we will see something different from initial appearances. The intense panic that virtually every cancer patient experiences is actually the mind projecting its fears about the unknown future. Think about it, and understand this truth: Panic is caused by the mind. It's an assumption. It is not based on material fact.

Our fear-filled thoughts do not necessarily determine our future. We have a choice. This is a profound healing insight.

What to do when you start to feel anxious emotions arising inside? Try to witness them. Just observe. You may want to give those emotions an image. View them, and yourself, in your mind's eye. Instead of putting yourself in the role of a victim who is hopelessly caught in a web of panic and despair, become the observer. By not engaging the mind in battle, by simply watching the emotions and letting go, your panic will soon subside.

For example, Gwen Clement said she gave her fears a name. She would catch herself becoming anxious and say, "Hey, Mr. Fear. What are you doing here? Get out of my life." Then she would replace that fear with a short prayer of gratitude. "Thank you, God, for giving me long life."

I encourage you to do the same, to develop your version of speaking to your fears, to literally tell them to go away. Then always end by imagining yourself as a victor. Give yourself an image of a competent and confident person who is about to make some very important choices. Clear decision-making can and will be yours.

## An Important Thing You Can Do

Sit down. Take a deep breath. Say out loud, "Cancer does not mean death." Observe your emotions. Detach by separating who you are as a person from the emotional panic you may be feeling. You are not uncontrolled fear even though you may be experiencing fear. Understand that difference. Then immediately read and act on the next two steps in this book.

# #2

---

# TAKE CHARGE

Who is the most important person on your cancer recovery team? Some people believe it is their surgeon. Others believe it is their oncologist. Some choose the medical or diagnostic technicians, others the nurses, and still others choose their spouse.

But the most important person on your cancer recovery team is you! You are the one who is ill. It is you who must work to get well again. You are the character of central importance. And you need to put yourself in charge.

Millions of cancer patients surrender leadership of their recovery program way too often and way too willingly. Elizabeth Smalley, a thirty-eight-year-old housewife, was diagnosed with breast cancer. Her treatment was not progressing as expected, and the side effects depleted her. It all left Elizabeth understandably discouraged. Her doctor kept assuring her, "We're doing all we can. Trust me."

Following an especially difficult week, Elizabeth asked herself, "Do I accept the course of this treatment or do I try something new?" She called and made an appointment at a comprehensive cancer center that was a four-hour drive from her home. Doctors there recommended a different treatment program. Elizabeth took back that recommendation to her home doctor for implementation. "Personally taking charge was my turning point," explained a healthy Elizabeth four years after her bold and assertive decision.

Survivors take charge. View yourself as the manager of a baseball team or whatever organizational analogy you like. This is your cancer recovery team. The team's mission is to get you well again. You'll want a strong starting pitcher; many times that is a nutritionist or an oncologist. And you'll need many other team members: a catcher, infielders, outfielders. Equate these with specialists. You, the manager, choose the team that is on the field at any given moment.

Traditionally, consumers play a passive role in the health-care system, going along with virtually whatever doctors and allied health-care professionals recommend. We're encouraged to consent. Is that why we're called "patients"? This passive attitude does not serve you well. Decide you will take charge now!

## An Important Thing You Can Do

Evaluate your team. Who are the players? Who is managing this team? Is it a one-person show? How many more people could be helping? Are the team members working for you? Do some seem to be working against you? One woman remarked, "Every time I go to the doctor, I feel like I am in enemy territory." If you feel that way, you need to make a substitution. Remember: You are in charge!

# #3

# ASK
# YOUR
# DOCTOR
# THESE
# QUESTIONS

It is critically important for you to clearly understand your diagnosis and the proposed treatment. The doctor who diagnosed you should answer the following questions. Record the answers:

1. Precisely what type of cancer do I have?_____
   Breast cancer patients: Ask if the cancer is invasive, what the hormone receptor tests show, and what the HER2 status is.
2. Has the cancer spread beyond the primary site? If so, where?

_____

3. What tests did you use to determine this diagnosis?

_____

4. May I have a copy of the pathology report?

_____

5. Is there any indication that a second pathology report is needed?

_____

6. Are you recommending additional tests? What are you looking for with each test?

_____

_____

7. How certain are you that the tests and the resulting diagnosis are accurate?

_____

8. What are my treatment options?

_____

_____

_____

9. Which one(s) do you recommend? (Record these recommendations in precise detail.)

_____

10. Whom would you recommend for a second opinion?

_____

You should detect an edge of skepticism in these questions. As a cancer patient you are a consumer. The decision process regarding who will prescribe and administer your treatment is not that much different from any other major purchase. But the consequences of your decisions are radically different from those involved in buying an automobile, for example.

You have the right, even the responsibility, to ask questions of your doctor just as you would with any consumer purchase. Evaluate those answers more closely than any major purchase you have ever made. Your options and choices for the best treatment will then become clearer.

Cancer survivors are consumer activists. They ask. Become an activist!

## An Important Thing You Can Do

Obtain answers to the preceding questions today! Record the answers in your Wellness and Recovery Journal. Ask the same questions again at the time you obtain your second opinion.

# #4

---

## GET
## TWO
## SECOND
## OPINIONS

Obtain second opinions from two board-certified oncologists, or cancer specialists. This is a critically important step that is not to be overlooked. If at all possible, the second opinions should be completed prior to starting any treatment program.

Whom you consult is also critically important. The second opinions should come from a multidisciplinary team. Typically you will want to speak to a surgeon, a radiation oncologist, and a medical oncologist. Why? Each will look at your case through his or her own training and experience. A radiation oncologist will typically say, "Radiation." A medical oncologist will typically say, "Chemotherapy." Let each of the oncologists know you will be talking to the other specialist. This knowledge alone will act as another checkpoint of control.

Additionally, the second opinion doctors need to be independent of each other as well as not in a working partnership, formal or informal, with the doctor who made the initial diagnosis. Look for different hospital and medical group affiliations. Many people travel to major cancer centers to obtain them. Second opinion consultations are that important.

Do not be fearful that a request for a second opinion might alienate your doctor. Second opinion consultations are standard procedure; your doctor makes such referrals every day. Ask the doctor who made the initial diagnosis, or a member of the staff, for a complete transcript of your medical records. Then take the records with you, or have them sent ahead. I prefer to personally hand the records to the consulting staff. It eliminates the chance of lost pages and delays.

The cost of obtaining at least one second opinion is reimbursed by virtually all insurance programs. Even if you're not covered, get the second opinions. Don't let cost stand in the way of obtaining some of the most important advice of your life.

"I had a second opinion all right," explained Katherine Gerhardt, a fifty-five-year-old insurance office manager and grandmother, describing her experience with breast cancer. "The second opinion came from another surgeon who shared offices with the first. They both said "radical" (mastectomy) was the way to go. And to this day I wonder if I would have been better off with a lumpectomy and radiation."

Katherine's second opinion experience could have been improved in two ways. First, she would have been better served by consulting with an oncologist. These specialists diagnose and treat cancer every working day. They can be expected to have the most up-to-date information on treatment options for each type and stage of cancer. Both surgeons Katherine consulted were general surgeons who dealt with a variety of illnesses, not just cancer.

Second, Katherine would have been better served by consulting with a second opinion doctor not associated with the first. Her surgeons were located in the same building and just down the hall from her family doctor.

These associations are a little-discussed but potentially important issue to patients. Doctors who are friends, office mates, business associates, or in a junior position within a medical practice may find it difficult to challenge the diagnoses or recommended treatment programs of associates. All sorts of relationships exist that may influence decisions. "We were in the middle of rene-gotiating the lease," said Robert, a young oncologist who rented office space from another oncologist. "We were meeting that very afternoon to discuss rents. I didn't want to offend my landlord when he sent me a patient for a second opinion consultation. So I just agreed with his treatment recommendations."

That experience may seem improbable, but the story is un-fortunately true. The best safeguard is to seek second opinions from board-certified oncologists with different specialties, who are affiliated with different practices, at different hospitals, and perhaps even live in different cities.

It puzzles me why so many cancer patients are fearful of ask-ing for a second opinion. When I have inquired, the typical re-sponse is, "No one told me to ask," or, "I don't want to offend my doctor."

Obtaining a second opinion in no way implies that the initial diagnosis is incorrect, that the suggested treatment is inappropri-ate, or that you lack confidence in the physician. On a subject as important as this, you simply deserve to have the benefit of more than one person's thinking. Your second opinion search also puts you in touch with other doctors, giving you options and helping you decide which medical team will actually administer your treatment program.

John was a sixty-two-year-old accountant diagnosed with colon cancer. His primary care doctor suggested John consult with a surgeon. The day John's second set of test results came back from the lab, the surgeon called John, confirmed the initial diagnosis, and said, "I've scheduled you for surgery. Be at the hospital by six-thirty tomorrow morning." Fortunately, John had the courage to say "slow down" and went about obtaining another second opinion consultation from a board-certified medical oncologist.

The second opinion oncologist independently confirmed the initial diagnosis. In fact, he also recommended surgery, just as John was initially advised. John returned to his surgeon only to be greeted with sarcasm: "I told you so. What's the matter? Didn't you trust me?" John walked out of that doctor's office, found another surgeon, and today is in excellent health. The lessons: Second opinions are critical. And you do not have to accept intimidation or arrogance.

## An Important Thing You Can Do

Make your second opinion appointments today. This is one of the most important things you can do. *Do not overlook this step*. Act now! Pick up the phone. Make the appointments.

# # 5

# BECOME AN
# E-PATIENT

Turn to the Internet to research your diagnosis, understand all your treatment options, and connect with other patients similarly diagnosed. Here's a handful of the best resources:

Cancer Recovery Foundation. www.cancerrecovery.org. The award-winning resource for integrated cancer care. Helps you mobilize body, mind, and spirit to get well and stay well. Analysis of conventional, complementary, and alternative treatment options. Extensive nutritional guidance. Suggested exercise regimens. Attitude builders. Support, both individual and groups, online and via telephone. Spiritually inclusive.

Oncolink. www.oncolink.edu. The top medically based cancer Website. Managed by the University of Pennsylvania, this site provides clinical information in understandable language. Comprehensive information about all the specific types of cancers, their conventional treatment options, and research news.

Komen (Susan G.) for the Cure. www.komen.org The world's largest breast cancer fund-raising organization. Understandable information on diagnosis, second opinions, treatment options, and survivorship.

## An Important Thing You Can Do

Contact www.cancerrecovery.org today. If you do not have computer access, call us toll-free in any of the countries we are located:

| | |
|---|---|
| Australia | +61(0)2 9929 5156 |
| Canada | 1-866-753-0303 |
| France | +33(0)1 44 39 1953 |
| Germany | +49(0) 69 66 40 880 |
| United Kingdom | 1-020 8249 6054 |
| United States | 1-800-238-6479 |

Hold yourself accountable for an in-depth knowledge of your diagnosis, treatment options, and self-help action plan.

# #6

---

# RETHINK
# THE
# STATISTICS

As you conduct your research into treatment options, you will invariably discover cancer recovery statistics that detail cancer incidence, mortality, and five-year survival rates. Do not let these statistics paralyze you. Your response to them is critical.

Statistics measure populations. They can be interpreted in a great many ways. But statistics do not determine any individual case, including yours.

Just after my second surgery, I received a booklet filled with numerical tables, statistics, and graphs on all types of cancers. Of course I felt compelled to read all the information on lung cancer. The numbers on metastatic lung cancer were not promising. As I reflected on what I read, I felt frightened, depressed, and filled with despair, certain of my fast-approaching death.

Several days later I looked again at those statistics and realized that many people do survive. "What did the survivors do?" I wondered. "How can I learn from them?"

No matter how difficult your situation, realize that there is no type of cancer that does not have some rate of survival. This is a significant fact, and it is cause for reasonable hope. The question now becomes, "What can I do to maximize my chances of getting on the right side of these statistics?"

With this book you have already begun to tap into the answers.

## An Important Thing You Can Do

Interpret statistics as indications of progress. Determine to act with the conviction that you will be counted among the "survivor statistics."

# #7

## UNDERSTAND YOUR CONVENTIONAL TREATMENT OPTIONS

In addition to the information you generate from your own research, you should expect your oncologist to carefully explain which type of conventional treatment(s) is recommended for your type and stage of cancer. The options will typically fall into one or a combination of three primary treatment modalities:

- Surgery: removal of the tumor
- Radiation: exposure to X-rays or radium
- Chemotherapy: the use of cytotoxic chemicals

Surgery is the most frequently employed cancer treatment. It is best used when the cancer is small and has not moved to other parts of the body. Radiation therapy is employed in approximately one-half of all cancer cases. It is often used in combination with other treatment options, for example either before or after surgery. Chemotherapy is most often used when the cancer has spread or when the diagnosis is a systemic-type cancer. It is often used in combination with radiation therapy and surgery to control tumor growth.

Three other types of conventional medical treatment modalities are being used more frequently:

- Hormonal: employs or manipulates bodily hormones
- Immunotherapy: enhancing the body's own immune function
- Investigative: experimental programs

Hormonal treatment is used in cancers that depend on hormones for their growth. Hormones are either removed, added, or their production is blocked through drugs or surgery that removes the hormone-producing gland. Immunotherapy includes the cytokines, like the family of interleukins and interferons, and is an attempt to boost or restore the body's natural defense system. Many people believe immunotherapies will soon comprise a fourth widely accepted treatment modality. At this writing, their scientific efficacy is yet to be established. Investigative protocols are experimental. They are typically the last choice.

As you evaluate your conventional treatment options, please carefully consider some of my personal observations from over two decades of helping patients make informed choices:

1. While surgery is the most common form of conventional treatment, dozens of types of cancer diagnosis do not indicate surgery. Many patients panic when they are told their cancer is "inoperable." If you have been told that your cancer in inoperable, do not despair. Recognize that inoperable does not equate with incurable!

2. If your oncologist suggests surgery, and you concur, the decision as to who actually performs the procedure is yours. Your choice of surgeons is important. You're more likely to get a well-qualified surgeon if you choose one who is a fellow of the Ameri-

can College of Surgeons and who is also board certified in his or her field. Only about half of practicing surgeons are board certified, so be sure to ask.

*Special note to premenopausal breast cancer patients:*
You typically have some flexibility on the timing of your surgery. Scientific evidence is mounting that fewer breast cancer recurrences are reported among women who choose to have their surgery during the luteal phase of the menstrual cycle, i.e., fourteen to thirty days following the onset of menstruation. Except for one Canadian study that suggested day 8 to be the optimal time, research shows surgery performed in the latter half of the menstrual cycle results in the fewest recurrences. Ask your surgeon for the most up-to-date research information prior to scheduling. You may have to assert yourself here; most surgeries are scheduled at the convenience of the surgeon and/or the hospital.

3. Thoroughly understand chemotherapy. Before you say yes to chemotherapy, ask to see proof, such as scientific papers and reports, on the effectiveness of the treatment being offered. Examine the hard evidence that the suggested chemotherapy protocol actually *cures, extends life, or improves quality of life.* Those are the three "outcomes" against which you must measure all treatments—conventional, experimental, complementary, and alternative.

If your clinician uses the terms "response" or "tumor response" or "reduce the tumor burden" or "achieve a remission," these represent different standards. These terms mean shrinkage or stopping the progression of the cancer. None of these terms are synonymous with "cure." A cure actually requires that your body fight the cancer on a cellular level and that your immune system maintain a disease-free state. To maximize your opportunity for such a response, I encourage you to follow as many of the health-enhancing, life-enriching principles in this book as possible.

Study the chemotherapy treatment option in depth. Do your

own research. Ask about both short-term and long-term side effects. Request the names and phone numbers of long-term survivors who were treated with similar regimens. Ask for their experience and analysis. Know exactly what you can expect— and not expect—chemotherapy to accomplish. Once you possess that information, you are in a position to make a truly informed decision. (See Appendix A, page 183, for a more detailed discussion of chemotherapy options.)

4. The administration of chemotherapy is not an exact science. Ask your oncologist about chemotherapy sensitivity (in vitro) testing. Here, samples of your tissue are chemically analyzed in laboratory tests to determine interaction with different agents. In about a week, your oncologist will receive a report establishing which drugs are not likely to work as well as the most active agents. The net effect is a personalized treatment program optimized before you begin.

5. Chemotherapy may be in pill form, to be taken by mouth, or it may be in liquid form and injected into a muscle or, most commonly, given through a vein. The drugs may be administered in a daily, weekly, or monthly program for periods ranging from a few months to a lifetime. Side effects, once the fear of all patients, are now being more effectively controlled. Refer in this book to #36, "Minimize Treatment Side Effects," for helpful things you can do to control uncomfortable side effects.

6. Radiation therapy is most often administered by means of an external beam machine. Internal radiation is becoming more common, where radioactive material is surgically implanted into or on the area to be treated. This procedure requires precision. You will maximize your opportunity for receiving excellent care if you choose a physician who is certified by the American Board of Radiology. Ask.

All cancers are treatable. Even in cases where the cancer is advanced, experimental investigative programs are available. If your cancer is not responding to conventional treatment, ask about hormonal treatment and biological response modifiers. Especially consider the many complementary and alternative programs described in this book. You are entitled to understand the full range of treatments available. From that understanding, you will have the knowledge and power to make the most intelligent treatment decisions.

Once again, conventional treatment has its important place. In interviews with thousands of cancer survivors, over 96 percent stated they initiated a course of conventional therapy. It is a myth that cancer survivors turn exclusively to alternative, nontraditional cancer treatments in large numbers. In the late 1980s, a Food and Drug Administration study estimated that 40 percent of cancer patients used unconventional treatments. That may be true; in fact, I believe the number may now be much higher, perhaps 60 percent. But survivors do not give up the traditional treatments. They integrate complementary and alternative practices into a comprehensive recovery program. That is what the guidance in this book is all about.

*A final thought on conventional treatment options:*

Please clearly understand this point: the vast majority of survivors select a conventional program using surgery, chemotherapy, or radiation, often in combination, as the foundation of their treatment. Survivors then supplement this conventional approach with many of the ideas presented in this book. I recommend you implement a conventional medical treatment program based on your own research and your own strong belief. However, I also believe your treatment is not complete until you initiate a comprehensive and integrated cancer recovery program. Given our current levels of understanding, this integration represents your very best opportunity for surviving cancer.

## An Important Thing You Can Do

Ask your oncologist to explain the specific treatment options available to you in the areas of surgery, radiation, and chemotherapy. Ask also about hormonal, immunotherapy, and investigative programs. Ask for his or her recommendation. Then check these recommendations against the "What to Expect in Treatment" section of the Cancer Recovery Foundation Website, www.cancerrecovery.org. Record this information in your Wellness and Recovery Journal. *Do not* give your approval for treatment just yet. First, more work remains to be completed.

# #8

## GAUGE YOUR CONFIDENCE IN YOUR MEDICAL TEAM

Few patients have any objective way to judge whether their surgeons, oncologists, or other medical professionals have technical competence. We can consider our medical team's education and professional certifications, and the experiences of other patients. But few of us can evaluate, with technical accuracy, whether a particular doctor will be able to address our specific case with success. We can, however, make subjective assessments, the kind of judgments that can be enormously important in our recovery journey. We can intuitively gauge our confidence level.

Ann Simmons, a highly successful insurance executive, was diagnosed with ovarian cancer. By the time it was discovered, the metastasis was significant and the prognosis poor. Ann interviewed seven different oncologists. She went to them with her pathology report and diagnosis in hand and simply asked, "Assuming this diagnosis is correct, what would you have me do?"

The answers she received were actually fairly predictable and consistent. That was reassuring. But what was more comforting was one oncologist's interpersonal skills. He listened. He asked questions to determine Ann's confidence in a procedure. Based on Ann's answers, and her confidence level, he offered his recommendations. Ann chose this doctor.

Ann's analysis was based not so much on any objective measures of technical competence but on her intuition, her belief in a person and a recommended program. She followed that intuition.

I believe you can trust your intuition provided you double-check it. To be sure, an excellent bedside manner can seldom make up for a lack of training, knowledge, and technical expertise. But survivors have repeatedly told me there is a direct correlation between the confidence one has in one's health-care team and the probability of recovery. Communication skills shape that confidence level. You are seeking a balance here.

## An Important Thing You Can Do

Evaluate your confidence level following an encounter with members of your medical team. This is particularly important when you are being asked to make treatment decisions. If you harbor more doubt than assurance toward your health-care providers and their recommendations, it is time to change either your confidence level or your team.

---

*Be sure you are approaching this work at a comfortable pace. I suggest you take a break now and reflect on this important step. Continue your work after you have rested.*

# #9

# CONVICTION VERSUS WISHFUL THINKING

Following an ovarian cancer diagnosis, Elaine Bothwell, a busy mother and community volunteer, was told by her oncologist that an aggressive course of chemotherapy, one that would require hospitalization, was recommended.

Elaine deeply feared chemotherapy. Still vivid in her memory was her mother-in-law's agonizing death from cancer. The side effects of treatment were much worse than the illness. Elaine vowed at that time if she were ever diagnosed with cancer she would never have chemotherapy. Now she faced precisely the situation she feared most.

Elaine went in search of nontraditional treatments. Among others, she consulted a naturopath who suggested metabolic therapy, a combination of detoxification, herbs, and hyperthermia (the use of heat) to help destroy cancer cells. While this program sounded minimally toxic and noninvasive, Elaine now feared she was getting too far away from conventional medical care.

Then Elaine went to another medical oncologist. After she explained her fears and her search, this doctor recommended the use of hormones. Elaine was assured that hormonal therapy was typically less toxic than chemotherapy and in most cases generated far fewer side effects. But the hormone treatment was not as highly recommended as the original and more effective chemotherapy program.

Torn between these three different approaches, Elaine realized that the treatment she was most convinced would work was a combination of two. Through sheer persistence she was able to find a cancer treatment center that combined fractionated-dose chemotherapy with hyperthermia. On her own, she adopted a nutritional supplementation program that included the herbs. She decided to hold the hormone treatment in reserve.

Elaine's choice of treatment is clearly not the answer for everyone. But following one's conviction is an important element of nearly every successful treatment program. Today, nineteen years after her initial diagnosis, Elaine's cancer remains in remission, and she leads a full and happy life.

"I wanted conviction from my doctor," said Bill Follett, a colon cancer survivor. "I looked him right in the eyes and asked, 'Is this treatment just the conventional thinking, Doctor? Or can you show me the hard data to back up your recommendation?' When he reviewed the published research, it seemed surgery followed by chemotherapy was my best bet."

## An Important Thing You Can Do

Before you commit to a treatment program, take the time to ask yourself some critical questions: "Do I hold the belief that this is the right thing to be doing?" "Am I just taking the path of least resistance?" If you don't believe in it, resist! Find a treatment program that you can follow with conviction.

# #10

---

# REFLECT
## ON THE
## TREATMENT
## DECISION

If you've carefully read each step up to this point, you'll realize that you've simply been gathering information about treatment options. You have not yet made any treatment decisions. Now it is time to systematically review your treatment options one last time prior to crossing this Rubicon.

First, compare. Are you receiving consistent information from:

- The doctor who made the initial diagnosis?
- The oncologists whom you consulted for your second opinions?
- The recommendations you found through your independent research?

You should expect to see a reasonable consistency in the recommendations you receive from these sources. Most treatment variances should relate to differences in levels of toxicity and degrees of invasiveness. If there is fundamental agreement, your decision-making process will probably be straightforward.

If the recommendations are inconsistent, then your information gathering is not complete. When you receive mixed signals, it is a certain sign to obtain a third qualified and independent opinion. This is time and money wisely spent.

Several providers in the oncology community have criticized me for this suggestion. Their objections have included: "The differences in treatment that you'll find are actually very minor." "Most patients cannot afford the cost." "You're just losing valuable time in receiving treatment." I disagree.

In all but the very rare case, the few days spent in gaining third or fourth opinions are well worth the wait. We can all find the funds if necessary. As a patient you are after the very best treatment. You should expect a consistency of recommendations, if not a consensus.

Terry Bartholomew is a forty-seven-year-old man from Indiana who was diagnosed with lymphoma. He obtained eight different opinions before agreeing to a program of treatment. Terry's determination to find the best has proven wise, and today he is alive and well.

Terry's experience points to an objection patients often raise: "But my insurance won't cover a third or fourth opinion." My response is, "Find a way." I was only too glad to pay for the services of qualified medical experts who would help determine the best course of treatment for me. Develop a similar attitude. Don't let insurance coverage limits determine this issue. Borrow the money or even seek out a free clinic. There is nothing more important in your life at this moment.

Once you attain clarity and conviction in terms of the medical treatment, another evaluation needs a second reflective look. Are you comfortable with the people who will give you treatment and the place where the treatment will be administered?

June Callas, a single mother in her fifties, had ovarian cancer. The treatment program in which she had the most confidence was recommended by doctors at a cancer center that was located more than an hour's commute over busy California freeways. She was expected to visit the center weekly while undergoing treatment. The commute was a problem. June didn't want to drive in rush-hour traffic; a friend or family member would have to act as chauffeur. She also didn't feel completely safe in the part of the city where the treatment center was located.

June expressed her concerns about the drive and her physical safety to the supervising oncologist. The doctor's response was compassionate and understanding. He was able to make arrangements at a hospital only ten minutes from June's apartment. She could receive her weekly treatments there and visit the cancer center just once a month. To this day, June believes the change in location was an important part of her successful recovery.

Does the recommended treatment program truly have your conviction? Are you convinced that the recommendations are the finest? Conviction implies a sense of certainty. While there are no guarantees, your treatment program and the people who administer it should elicit a strong degree of certainty that this is the right path to be taking at this time.

Cancer Recovery Foundation has helped thousands of cancer patients walk through this treatment option analysis. Invariably a question arises: "What about all the alternative approaches? I really haven't checked them out." We have consistently recommended this strategy: First, explore the conventional treatment options. Surgery, radiation, and chemotherapy are the basis for the overwhelming majority of survivor success stories.

If the conventional treatment methods hold no real promise, then analyze both the investigative options as well as the complementary and alternative therapies.

With all the options, integrate improved diet and nutritional supplementation, plus the psychosocial and psychospiritual techniques. Mobilize body, mind, and spirit. I believe that a physician who withholds this integrated treatment approach is no longer offering an informed medical opinion.

Allow yourself time to reflect on these important decisions. Don't be pressured by anyone to hurry a decision. When the treatment recommendations are consistent, the people who administer the treatment have your confidence; you understand the importance of integrating body, mind, and spirit; and you can say with conviction that this is what you should be doing now. Then, and only then, are you ready to go to the next step.

## An Important Thing You Can Do

Consult your notations in your Wellness and Recovery Journal. Thoughtfully, carefully, systematically, reflect on your treatment decision. Take another break. Reflect . . . again.

# #11

## DECIDE!

There is power in decision.

The cancer journey is made up of both little decisions and big decisions. Your treatment program is a big one. In many ways it will determine the direction of your entire life. Now is the time to decide.

Decision is the spark that ignites action. Until a decision is reached, nothing happens.

Making decisions like this takes courage. But there is power in facing the fact that you have cancer, then carefully doing your homework, and finally choosing a course of action. Without exercising your courage, the problem will remain forever unaddressed.

Decide! Do not straddle the fence or make a partial decision. This is the time to take a firm stand on one side or another. Make a full commitment.

Yes, you will monitor your decision. You will keep your options open, of course. But now is the moment to say, "This is how we will climb the mountain! Now let's get started!"

Decision frees us from many of the uncertainties caused by fear, doubt, and anxiety. Yes, there is risk. But there is greater risk in making no decision, hoping that all will magically be well.

Decide. You've done the work. This is not blind chance. This decision is the culmination of careful and sustained inquiry. Now is the time for action.

Decision awakens the spirit. Do you feel a new awakening? Do you sense that part of you is springing to life? Nourish that spirit. Cherish it. It is the life force inside you working for you, helping you get well again.

Decide. The decision comes first, the results follow. Today is the day. Now is the hour. This is the moment! Decide!

## An Important Thing You Can Do

Now, make the treatment decision. Appreciate the power of your commitment. Be optimistic. Decide! Inform your team of your choice.

# #12

## GIVE ONLY INFORMED CONSENT

All treatment decisions should be made—must be made—with the informed consent of the patient or patient's guardian. This means you need to know in detail, in terms you can clearly understand, all the risks entailed in any procedure involving surgery, anesthesia, radiation therapy, chemotherapy, or a similar medical encounter.

You'll be asked to sign a consent form. Do not sign a blank consent form. Make certain that the exact procedure is described and that you fully understand it. You have the right to set limits on these documents. You can cross out statements to which you do not consent. For example, I drew a line through the section of my consent form that asked my permission to videotape the operation for the removal of my lung.

You have the right to refuse treatment. An adult who is mentally competent can refuse treatment even if it may result in death. Nancy was a young woman who was pregnant. Even though she was advised to go ahead with treatment for lung cancer, she felt so strongly about the potential harm to her unborn child that she elected to postpone treatment until after her delivery. She exercised her right to refuse consent.

You need to understand clearly and completely all to which you are consenting. Gary Nadine, a retired pilot who made his home in Oregon, recognized that something was wrong with his health when he began to feel weak all the time. In six months he lost more than twenty pounds without dieting. "I just wasn't hungry," he said. "And I felt like I had a low-grade fever all the time." Then Gary became aware of swelling in his abdomen.

Finally he went to his doctor, who ordered a variety of tests. There was a complete physical examination, the most thorough he had ever experienced. Then chest X-rays, CAT scans, a blood workup, urine tests, and more. After consulting with other specialists, the doctor finally told Gary he had Hodgkin's disease.

Gary signed a consent form that said "laparotomy," thinking that he was giving permission for a biopsy. "The way it was presented," said Gary, "this seemed like just another test to determine, with more certainty, the extent of the disease. The doctor told me they needed to know where the cancer had spread. I thought it was no big deal and that I'd be out of the hospital the next day."

In fact, it was a big deal and Gary was not fully informed. A laparotomy is a surgical procedure that allows the doctors to explore the entire abdominal area. It is major surgery that should only be done by a team of experienced surgeons. Because of complications and infections, Gary's hospital stay lasted two and a half weeks. It left him with significant scars and lasting discomfort.

While Gary technically, even legally, gave consent to the procedure, in his mind he gave his okay for something much different. "I should have asked," lamented Gary. "But it seemed like no big deal."

Your doctor is obligated to inform you fully of any procedure to which you are being asked to give consent. This means explaining to you the procedure's purpose and risks, other alternatives, and the risk involved in not having the procedure. Don't be intimidated by the medical lingo. Make certain you get this information in language you understand. More important, make certain you ask detailed questions prior to giving any consent. Don't tolerate a physician's attitude that your concerns are unwelcome. If he or she is condescending or overly impatient, find another doctor. And be certain to include on your list of questions, "Why is this procedure absolutely necessary?"

## An Important Thing You Can Do

Ask your physician—not an associate, not an assistant, and not a nurse—to describe clearly the risks involved in your tests and treatment. Compare the risks to the expected benefits.

# #13

## BELIEVE IN YOUR TREATMENT PROGRAM

Excited belief is one of the great intangibles in a successful cancer treatment program. It is a natural extension of your conviction about your integrated treatment decisions. And it is your personal responsibility to believe in, and even be excited about, your treatment program.

Rachael Katz and May Tyson both attended one of our Cancer Recovery seminars in Atlanta. Rachael is a Georgia homemaker who started a course of radiation following surgery for breast cancer. Her attitude toward treatment was, "I guess it's something I have to do."

May received virtually the same diagnosis about a month after Rachael. May also had surgery and a follow-up course of chemotherapy. But her attitude was totally different from Rachael's: "I saw those chemicals as a great healing agent, something coming into my body to make me well. I welcomed my chemotherapy with open arms!"

Today May is free of cancer. Rachael continues to struggle.

Cancer survivors develop a confidence and an *excited belief* in their treatment programs that other patients do not possess. I am convinced that a direct correlation exists between belief in one's treatment and its effectiveness. My observations of the importance of belief in cancer treatment lead me to respect the awesome power of the mind and the human spirit in the cancer journey. I want to see you mobilize those resources in your own program.

Cassandra Pooley is a California wife, mother, and now retired elementary school teacher. After three years of remission, she had a recurrence of breast cancer including liver and bone metastasis. Her doctors gave her less than a year to live. "I knew I was at the crossroads," said Cassandra. "And when I learned that survivors held an excited belief about their treatment, I knew I had to change my expectations and get excited."

You can observe excited and expectant belief in survivor after survivor. I fully realize my observations are only anecdotal evidence and cannot stand up to scientific scrutiny. But I do believe this hypothesis is true. Cancer survival is a matter of involving both head and heart. I have seen beliefs and attitudes like May's and Cassandra's make the difference in hundreds of cases. To me the correlation between belief in treatment and effectiveness of treatment is very high.

Someday the scientific and medical communities will fully document the biological reality of this kind of optimism. In the meantime, I suggest you not enter the debate. Instead, learn from the survivors and develop an excited belief about your treatment.

## An Important Thing You Can Do

"Own" your treatment program. See it as a friend. Believe it is there to help you. Excited belief is what you seek.

# #14

## OVERCOME FATIGUE AND NAUSEA

Extreme fatigue is reported by nearly 90 percent of cancer patients both during and after treatment. Worse, getting more sleep or rest often does not relieve the fatigue. In fact, cancer-related fatigue is one of the most profound and distressing issues patients face. This unique type of fatigue can have dozens of causes, and for patients who have completed cancer therapy, fatigue is among their foremost concerns, second only to fear of disease recurrence.

What can be done? Moderate exercise is the number one treatment for fatigue. In patient after patient, exercise was found to mitigate fatigue and lead to more restful and predictable sleep. You'll find more information on this important thing to do in section 26 of this book.

In addition, the popular dietary supplement ginseng appears to relieve fatigue and boost energy levels in people with cancer. Researchers studied 282 people with breast, colon, and other types of cancer. They were randomly assigned to take 750 milligrams, 1,000 milligrams, or 2,000 milligrams of American ginseng or a placebo daily for eight weeks.

About 25 percent of those on the two highest doses reported their fatigue was "moderately or much better," compared with only 10 percent of those taking the lowest dose or the placebo. Also, energy levels were about twice as high in those taking the 1,000-milligram dose as those taking the placebo.

People taking the two highest doses also reported generally feeling better, with improvements in mental, physical, spiritual, and emotional well-being. And they said they were more satisfied with their treatment.

The researchers tested the Wisconsin species of American ginseng, which is different from Chinese ginseng and other forms of American ginseng sold in health food stores. The ginseng was powdered and given in capsule form. However, the question remains unanswered on interactions with some conventional medical treatments.

Next is nausea. One of the realities for about half of the cancer patients undergoing chemotherapy is nausea. While there are other side effects, including hair loss, fatigue, and the decreased ability of the body to make red and white blood cells and platelets, nausea is typically the most uncomfortable. It may or may not include vomiting. Most people can significantly improve this experience, but it takes some experimentation. Here are some suggestions:

- Ask your oncologist for antinausea medication. Compazine, Tigan, and Zofran are commonly prescribed. Try taking them thirty to sixty minutes before treatments.
- Use relaxation exercises. (See section 34.)
- Eat smaller meals more often. Try six daily meals.
- Emphasize low-fat foods, especially fresh fruits.
- Limit liquids taken with meals. Drink no liquids in the hour before meals and the hour following meals. But be sure to take in enough liquids at other times. If you choose chemotherapy, your oncologist will tell you to drink more liquids to ensure good urine flow and minimize problems with the liver, kidneys, and bladder.

- Clear, cool liquids are recommended. Iced green tea, ginger ale, clear broths, popsicles, or apple juice ice cubes are worth trying. Take all liquids slowly.
- Eat dry food such as crackers, toast, or popcorn—especially at the start of the day or at the first sign of nausea. Sorry, no butter on the popcorn.
- Eat salty foods. Avoid overly sweet foods.
- Do not lie down for two hours after eating. You can rest sitting up. Or if you simply must stretch out, prop a couple of pillows under your head to gain elevation.
- Sometimes loose clothing or fresh air will help in nausea control.
- Ask your pharmacist about Travel-Eze or Seaband antinausea wrist bands.
- Drink ginger root tea steeped with peppermint.
- Goldenseal root may be helpful.
- Try hypnosis. Several small clinical trials have shown significant reductions in nausea and vomiting versus no hypnotherapy.

## An Important Thing You Can Do

Experiment. Clearly, there is no one-size-fits-all answer to fatigue and nausea. You'll need to try the suggested ideas. They have proven successful for many other cancer patients. They may be just the answer you have been searching for.

# #15

---

# MAKE
# THE MOST
# OF YOUR
# APPOINTMENTS

Free and open communication between you and your health-care team is one of the most important aspects of your cancer recovery journey. You need to stay informed. You want feedback. But seldom is this information volunteered. You'll have to ask for it.

Wise patients bring a list of questions to virtually every medical appointment. If you have continuing or new symptoms, ask about them. If you are experiencing side effects, ask about them. Ask for further information about issues raised from your reading or from talking to other patients.

"My radiation technician started to tease me about all my questions," said a retired Minneapolis professor who was being treated for prostate cancer. "I'd walk in the room and she'd say, 'What's on your list today, Dr. Nelson?' But I was determined to participate fully, to be an active patient. So I didn't let her remarks bother me in the least."

Speak with total honesty to your doctor and the entire health-care team. They are not mind readers. Tell them your problems and ask for their opinions. Bring a family member with you if you have trouble being assertive. He or she can be your advocate. Many people are intimidated by their doctors. If you are one of these people, recognize it and act immediately to remove that needless hurdle. If you are having trouble understanding and absorbing medical information, bring a tape recorder. Then you'll be able to review explanations and instructions at your convenience.

In case this hasn't been emphasized enough by now, please understand that your ability to ask questions is one of your most significant points of power. When in doubt, write down your questions and then read them from your list.

One other insider's tip: If you truly want to make the most of your medical appointments, get in the habit of expressing your sincere gratitude to your medical team. One of a group of doctors at a large health-care system in Pittsburgh lamented to me, "We try so earnestly to help a patient. I wish once in a while they would simply say thank you." I clearly remember giving an appreciative hug to my oncologist. From that day forward I was treated like royalty in that office. Start showing your appreciation to these very important people in your life. Remember, they're people who respond to you just as you respond to them.

## An Important Thing You Can Do

In your Wellness and Recovery Journal, record both your medical questions and the answers you are given. Keep this information handy. Bring it to your appointments. If you rely on your memory or record your questions on bits of paper scattered here and there, you'll never obtain timely and accurate information.

Write a thank-you note to at least one person on your medical team following your next visit.

# #16

## MONITOR YOUR PROGRESS

As you continue your treatment program, you'll be given tests to determine how well it's working. Ask about the tests prior to agreeing to them. Then insist that the doctor share the results in the form of copies of your test reports.

It's uplifting to know that you are making progress. But even a report that is less encouraging can have a positive side. It should lead you to consider other forms of treatment. Many exist. If all standard therapies have been exhausted, ask about investigative treatments. Or look more seriously at the complementary and alternative choices.

It is your responsibility to monitor your treatment program. Don't wait. Ask.

### An Important Thing You Can Do

Ask your doctor how and when he or she will check the progress of your treatment. Write this information in your Wellness and Recovery Journal. Then be certain tests occur as scheduled.

# HEAL
## YOUR
# LIFESTYLE

I am frequently asked, "How much did conventional medicine contribute to your survival?" My answer has been the same for over a decade: 10–15 percent. In my estimation, personal lifestyle choices were absolutely the key reason I am alive today.

A Stanford University health newsletter estimated that lifestyle issues such as poor diet, lack of exercise, and unwise health habits accounted for 61 percent of premature deaths due to cancer. They estimated the proportional share of genetics was 29 percent, and medical treatments themselves were listed as contributing to 10 percent of cancer deaths. I believe these estimates are probably low.

The central point is obvious: lifestyle choices are critical in the cancer survival journey. These are under our control, a matter of intention, an issue of personal choice. Clearly, there is much we can do to help ourselves get well and stay well. Let's examine how literally millions of people have helped in their own healing.

# #17

# LIVE
# "WELL"

Make wellness a way of life. Wellness is a stance one chooses in order to maximize one's health—physically, emotionally, and spiritually. The goal is to achieve the highest level of well-being possible in each of these areas of life.

Wellness recognizes and acts on the fact that everything one thinks, says, does, feels, and believes has an impact on one's well-being.

Wellness can be chosen at any moment, in any circumstance. Wellness is possible with disability, regardless of physical condition.

For most people, "living well" typically means some major changes in lifestyle—in body, mind, and spirit.

We previously stated that cancer survivorship is a combination of head and heart. Conquering cancer demands that you reach beyond the physical issues of illness. Your mental, emotional, and spiritual health has a powerful effect on your well-being.

Kelly Liddle is a forty-eight-year-old account executive with a major investment management firm. He developed malignant melanoma. "I went through the surgery and radiation just as recommended," said Kelly. "But I knew the real problem. I wasn't taking care of myself." Kelly hadn't exercised for years. His diet and nutrition habits were deplorable. He despised his work, and his marriage was coming apart.

Like so many survivors, Kelly considered cancer his wake-up call. "I realized my life was off course. And I knew it was up to me to change."

Similar sentiments are expressed by many survivors of cancer. They see illness as a message to make life changes. Kelly went on to reflect, "When I quit my job and opened a floral shop, my entire life started to heal. Cancer has actually been very good for me."

Living well, intentional choice, exercising the decision to take personal responsibility for one's total well-being—this is common talk among cancer survivors. It's whole-person wellness, a triumphant way of living without conditions.

*Without conditions* means that although wellness may be obscured by illness, it is a matter of personal choice whether wellness will be destroyed by illness. *Without conditions* means it is possible to discover high-level emotional and spiritual wellness in the very midst of life-threatening illness. The decision to "live well" is significant and profound. Never again will your well-being be a static state measured simply by the lack of negative physical symptoms.

My friend, I want to help you catch this vision for your health and your life. Join me. Let's make wellness our shared personal quest.

## An Important Thing You Can Do

Begin the wellness quest. Open your mind and spirit to whole-person wellness. In your Wellness and Recovery Journal, record one step you can take today to improve your greater well-being. Now act, doing what is clearly doable today. Determine to live life at a new and higher level of wellness no matter what.

# #18

# OPERATE
# UNDER
# NEW
# ASSUMPTIONS

Compare the assumptions behind orthodox health care with those behind whole-person wellness:

| Assumptions behind conventional health care | Assumptions behind whole-person wellness |
| --- | --- |
| 1. The patient is reliant upon the medical community. | 1. The patient has, or should develop, independence. |
| 2. The professional is the authority. | 2. The professional is a healing partner. |
| 3. Symptoms are treated, not investigated. | 3. The underlying causes are sought, plus the symptoms are treated. |
| 4. Specialized and concerned with body's subsystems. | 4. Unified and concerned with person's whole life. |
| 5. Body viewed as a series of mechanical functions. | 5. Body viewed as a changing system. |

6. Primary repairs made with surgery or drugs.

6. Intervention is minimal and appropriate. Noninvasive therapies are used when possible.

7. Pain and illness are purely negative.

7. Pain and illness are messages to value and act upon.

8. Mind and emotions are a secondary factor in health.

8. Mind and emotions are a major factor in health.

9. Body and mind are separate. Spirit has no health impact.

9. Body, mind, and spirit form one unit and always affect each other.

10. Disease prevention is largely environmental: not smoking, attention to diet, exercise, and rest.

10. Wellness means prevention plus wholeness: harmony in relationships, work, goals; a balance of body, mind, and spirit.

There is an important issue behind these assumptions. Your medical team will be helpful in addressing just one part of your cancer journey, the physical disease portion. Wellness encompasses far more. Whole-person well-being is our goal, and the responsibility for achieving it falls to each of us personally.

## An Important Thing You Can Do

Review the above assumptions. Circle those you believe to be true. Are you a traditionalist? Do you identify with the spirit of whole-person wellness? What does this analysis tell you to do differently? Which assumptions serve you best?

# #19

## SCHEDULE
## YOUR
## WELLNESS

All important tasks demand a schedule. And there is no more important work in your life right now than the work of getting well again.

The trouble is, most people keep putting off the work of wellness, thinking they will get to it later. And guess what? They seldom, if ever, get around to it. Or if they do, it's only after everything else that is "important" has been accomplished.

Develop the attitude that there is nothing more important in your life right now than your work of wellness. For the time being, your wellness efforts need to take priority over family, job, community or religious activities, and social obligations. Getting well is your new top priority; you need to incorporate the disciplines of wellness into your daily life.

I actually blocked out my week on a day planner. My typical weekday schedule looked like this while I was in the middle of recovery:

| | |
|---|---|
| 6:00 AM | Wake up |
| 6:15 | Exercise |
| 6:45 | Meditate |
| 7:00 | Shower, eat, and commute |
| 9:00 | Work |
| Noon | Lunch and meditate |
| 1:00 PM | Work |
| 4:30 | Commute |
| 5:30 | Meditate |
| 6:00 | Dinner |
| 7:00 | Family time |
| 9:00 | Read and meditate |
| 10:00 | Sleep |

Doctors' appointments were worked in as needed. During commutes I virtually always listened to wellness CDs. Weekends found me devoting even more time to study and meditation. Throughout the entire process, I became gentler with myself, demanding less in the way of outside activities and more in the way of self-care. I took control of my schedule and made the work of wellness my top priority.

## An Important Thing You Can Do

Start a new page in your Wellness and Recovery Journal. Plan a schedule for your week similar to mine. Minimize obligations that cause undue stress. Give ample "core time" to the wellness disciplines discussed in this book.

*After completing your schedule, I suggest you take a break from your wellness work. Start the next section tomorrow or after you have rested. In the meantime, give careful consideration to how you spend your time. Do you understand I am asking you to make wellness a way of life? For most people, this means a major lifestyle shift. Look within. Consider the evidence and the implications of these suggestions. Begin now to modify your schedule to meet your new wellness priorities.*

# #20

## ELIMINATE ACTIVE AND PASSIVE SMOKING

It totally mystifies me how some cancer patients can continue to use tobacco. John Everest had colon cancer. Following surgery, he started a course of chemotherapy. But do you think he quit smoking? No! "I don't have lung cancer," he'd say as he left our Cancer Recovery support sessions.

If I could communicate this any more strongly I would. Stop smoking! If you are a user, cut out any and all tobacco immediately. Cigarettes, cigars, chewing tobacco—all must go. There is no excuse, even nicotine addiction, that is sufficient to continue this harmful habit. Be clear: tobacco is putting cancer-causing chemicals into your body, something you do not need now or ever.

A family practitioner recently shared with me that he was not going to tell his patients to stop smoking. I was stunned and said, "What!?!?" "Some of them enjoy a cigarette," he said. "And besides, I don't want to offend them." My response was that smokers know they should quit, most want to quit and, far from being offended, they want their doctor to help them quit.

If you smoke, stop! The question is not whether you can quit. The question is whether you will quit. I know this firsthand. I started smoking when I was in my teens. There is no doubt that smoking directly contributed to my lung cancer just over twenty years later. In those twenty years I seriously tried to quit five or six times. Willpower alone didn't get the job done. A change in thinking did.

It started with changing my self-perception. I first went from perceiving myself as a smoker to seeing myself as a person who mistakenly chose the behavior of smoking. Seeing smoking as a behavior helped me detach emotionally and psychologically from the cigarettes. I began to perceive myself as a nonsmoker. A change in self-perception can work for you, too.

In addition to never smoking again, eliminate your exposure to passive smoking. A Finnish study revealed up to a one-third drop in circulating levels of vitamin C and other antioxidants after just thirty minutes of exposure to secondhand smoke. Always sit in the nonsmoking sections. Take charge. Support nonsmoking legislation in your area.

It has never been more important for you to maximize your health. Tobacco use and exposure to secondhand smoke have no place in the quest for wellness.

## An Important Thing You Can Do

Envision yourself as completely tobacco-free. Wean yourself with a nicotine patch if you must. But develop a self-image of being a nonsmoker deep in your spirit. And stay far, far away from tobacco users while they are smoking.

# #21

## ADOPT THIS NUTRITIONAL STRATEGY DURING TREATMENT

I was on the phone speaking to a man with metastatic prostate cancer. The subject quickly turned to nutrition. "What about your diet?" I asked. His reply was, "My doctor says I can eat anything I want."

No, dear readers, that may have been a medical opinion. But that was not an informed medical opinion. The days of "eat anything you want" are long behind. In fact, that philosophy may have contributed to the onset of this man's prostate cancer. It certainly detracts from maximizing one's total health and well-being.

Allow me some very straight talk: if you are determined to choose "eat anything" as your nutritional strategy, close this book now. This integrated cancer care program is not for you.

In the Road Map to Recovery section of this book, we briefly discussed nutritional strategy. Let's review. The most common nutritional shifts employed by cancer survivors are the following:

- Whole foods
- Foods low in fat, salt, and sugar

- Fresh vegetables, fresh fruits, and whole grains
- Adequate amounts of pure water

The single major dietary shift among cancer survivors is consuming foods that are less processed. If it is boxed or bottled or canned or packaged, the food comes under immediate scrutiny. Prepared foods, even when enriched, tend to deliver calories with less nutrition than their fresh counterparts. This means cancer survivors spend most of their grocery shopping time in the produce section of their local market.

Whole food means:

Fresh vegetables, fresh fruits, whole grains, whole grain pastas, brown rice, raw nuts, sprouted breads, and the like. See the cancer recovery shopping list in the next section.

Low fat, salt, and sugar means:

Good fats, like unsaturated fats, often classified into two groups: the omega-3s and the omega-6s. They come from extra virgin olive oil, sesame oil, seeds—especially flaxseed—and fatty fish.

Low salt means the right salt—sea salt or liquid aminos.

Low sugar means no added sugar. Sugar should come exclusively from whole food sources and then only in moderation.

Furthermore, please hear me on the importance of avoiding refined sugar. Scientists call sugar an "obligate glucose metabolizer." Loosely translated that means a "feeder." There exists significant evidence-based research pointing to sugar as doing two things that stand in the way of cancer recovery. First, sugar suppresses immune function. Second, it feeds cancer cells.

Diets high in sugar, and foods that turn into sugar when digested, cause blood sugar levels to rise. Once this spike is triggered, the body releases a hormone called insulin in an effort to bring the blood sugar levels back to normal. Understand this next key point: one of insulin's multiple functions is to promote cell growth—be that normal healthy cells or malignant cells. Therefore, the more insulin circulating in the body, the more opportunity for cancer cells to be fed, grow, and divide.

So, what can we actually do? Here's your new dietary guideline: "Whites out. Colors in."

"Whites out" mean no:

- White sugar
- White potatoes
- White rice
- White bread
- White pasta

All of these are simple carbohydrates that turn directly into sugar once ingested. Whites out! The days of a couple of teaspoons of sugar into your coffee or even raw or brown sugar onto your cereal are over. Stop eating refined sugar.

"Colors in" means to add:

Fresh vegetables of many colors including broccoli, kale, parsley, cabbage, romaine and leaf lettuce, spinach, peppers, cauliflower, beets, leeks, sweet potatoes, and more.

Fresh fruits of many colors including tomatoes (they are a fruit), apples, lemons, grapes, blueberries, and more. Just consume fruits in lesser quantities than vegetables. The sugar content in fruit is comparatively high.

There has never been a more important time in your life to eat well. Eating whole foods and those low in fat, salt, and sugar while emphasizing fresh fruits and vegetables is your new nutritional program.

## An Important Thing You Can Do

Wise nutrition is not a problem, it's a decision. So decide. Decide to eat healthfully, better than ever before in your entire life. See nutrition as of utmost importance, equal to or even more important than your medical treatment. Eating right starts with your decision. Decide!

# #22

# Shop for Nutritient-Dense Foods

The purpose of this section is to communicate in a clear, practical and useful manner the best food choices. The best way I know how to do this is by giving you a shopping list. All nutritional education is useless unless and until it is applied. A shopping list is a very good way to apply this knowledge.

The foods on this shopping list "pass the test." A passing grade is based on an analysis of a food's nutrient density. Nutrient density is a factor of vitamin, mineral, protein, fiber, and healthy fat(s) content, plus glycemic index and calories.

Shop from this "Nutrient-Dense" list:

**Vegetables**

___Broccoli
___Cabbage
___Peppers
___Tomatoes
___Carrots

**Fruits**

___Berries
___Oranges
___Red grapefruit
___Mangoes
___Apples

### Vegetables

___Leaf lettuce
___Cauliflower
___Onions
___Beets
___Asparagus
___Squash
___Pumpkin

### Fruits

___Cherries
___Apricots
___Cantaloupe
___Kiwis
___Pears
___Red grapes
___Watermelon

### Fish, Meat & Eggs

___Cod/flounder/haddock
___Tilapia/Mahi-mahi
___Salmon (wild)
___Tuna (canned/steaks)
___Trout (wild)
___Shrimp/Blue crab
___Sardines
___Eggs
___Skinless chicken breast
___Turkey breast

### Whole Grains & Breads

___Oats
___Barley
___Brown rice
___Flaxseed
___Buckwheat
___Spelt wheat
___Millet
___Amaranth
___Pita bread
___Wheat germ

### Legumes

___Black beans
___Garbanzo beans
___Kidney beans
___Navy beans
___Pinto beans
___Lentils
___Split peas

### Other

___Garlic
___Ginger
___Cinnamon
___Cayenne
___Stevia
___Green tea
___Curry

### Non-fat Dairy

___Yogurt
___Cottage cheese
___Soy milk

### Oils

___Extra virgin olive oil
___Sesame oil
___Non-fat vegetable spray

On the opposite end of the spectrum, there are several foods that clearly do not receive a passing grade. They deliver calories with few nutrients. This is the "No-Shop" list. During the cancer journey, do not put these foods in your shopping cart.

| | |
|---|---|
| \_\_\_Sugar | \_\_\_Liquor |
| \_\_\_Aspartame | \_\_\_Beer |
| \_\_\_Syrups | \_\_\_Wine |
| \_\_\_Hydrogenated fats | \_\_\_Soft drinks, regular |
| \_\_\_Lard | \_\_\_Soft drinks, diet |
| \_\_\_Margarine | \_\_\_Ice cream |
| \_\_\_Salami | \_\_\_Cookies |
| \_\_\_Hot dogs | \_\_\_Doughnuts |
| \_\_\_Bologna | \_\_\_Cake |
| \_\_\_Sausage | \_\_\_Boxed cereal |
| \_\_\_Bacon | \_\_\_Molasses |
| \_\_\_Smoked ham | \_\_\_Mayonaise |
| \_\_\_Pizza | \_\_\_Honey |

This does not mean you can never have another piece of pizza in your life. It does mean that this is the time in your life to "eat clean," meaning whole foods that are nutrient-dense and low in fat, salt, and sugar, with the clear emphasis on fresh vegetables, fresh fruits, and whole grains.

The good news is that there is an endless combination of menus based on nutrient-dense foods. So be creative. Experiment with your menus. You will be contributing to your health and well-being in a major way.

## An Important Thing You Can Do

If you are in the middle of the cancer journey, hold yourself accountable for shopping and eating from the approved "Nutrient-Dense" foods list.

# #23

## Drink Adequate Pure Water

Adequate pure water means six to eight glasses per day. Hopefully this is non-chlorinated pure spring water. But even tap water is better than being dehydrated.

Water is the basis of all bodily fluids, including digestive fluids, urine, lymph, and perspiration, as well as lubrication of our joints. Water is also essential for all cell activity, especially the transport of waste away from the cells and transport of nutrients to the cells.

Drink water. Coffee, tea, milk, soda, or alcoholic beverages do not count. Water. Pure water is the drink of choice.

It is an almost universal truth—people with cancer are dehydrated. Lack of water inhibits immune function, the most potent defense you have against cancer. The environment your cells live in is not blood, it is fluid. The lymph system, a key component of your immune system, is a fluid system requiring adequate water to function at its highest capacity.

Through natural elimination, perspiration, and even breathing, your body loses water daily. Fluid must be continually replaced in appropriate quantities for you to be optimally well.

I prefer water with no chlorine or fluorides. This is difficult to obtain from most municipal water systems. Even bottled water, especially if contained in plastic, is not a sure answer. Some research indicates that sunlight starts a chemical reaction in the plastic bottle that can result in carcinogens in the water.

How can you get pure water? I recommend a water purification system in your home or certified, chemical-free, spring-fed bottled water in glass containers.

## An Important Thing You Can Do

Drink eight cups of pure water each day.

# #24

# KNOW
# WHY
# YOU'RE
# EATING

Long-term dietary changes require more than shifts in our menus. Our food preferences are a factor of culture and habit. Our enjoyment of food is so much a part of our lives that any permanent change must involve not only *what* we eat but also *why* we eat.

On countless occasions we allow our frame of mind, rather than our body, to determine our food choices. Comfort foods to satisfy our emotions, to soothe our anger, frustration, worry, boredom, or guilt, are most often the culprit. Relief from emotional distress is easily accomplished by eating. When this happens we have linked diet to emotional fulfillment. This is dangerous territory.

We need a heightened awareness of why we eat. Many patients who embark on the cancer recovery journey develop an attitude that changing their diet is something they *have* to do. Too bad. I suggest you try an outlook that reflects the fact that a change in diet is something you *get* to do!

Eating with awareness is easily accomplished with the help of these practices:

- Don't keep any high-fat snack foods around the house where they will be a serious temptation.
- Make a rule of not eating in front of the television, where you don't pay attention to what or how much you eat.
- Don't eat so quickly that you can't enjoy your food. It takes about twenty minutes for the brain to realize that the stomach is full. Slow down. Take a break mid-meal.
- Reward appropriate eating behavior, but don't use comfort foods as the reward. If you've had a good week or have reached a wellness goal, treat yourself to a movie, a concert, or a new outfit. Don't punish imperfection, just don't reward yourself. Try again next week.
- Make each meal a pleasant experience. Stop eating on the run or while standing at the kitchen counter. Take time to put out a place setting. Offer a short affirmation or prayer of gratitude for each meal. You'll then be nurturing yourself emotionally and spiritually, as well as physically.

## An Important Thing You Can Do

Distinguish between a food craving, which is a psychological need, and hunger, which is the body's need for nourishment. Check your urge to eat the next time you see a food advertisement. A craving diminishes when you take on another activity. Go for a walk. Call a friend. Read a book. Then evaluate. Were you feeling a craving or hunger? Honor your hunger, not your craving. Eat with awareness!

# #25

# DETERMINE YOUR NUTRITIONAL SUPPLEMENT PROGRAM

**Fact:** Most cancer survivors believe in and use vitamin and mineral supplements.

**Fiction:** Vitamins are totally ineffective and should be avoided during cancer treatment.

The following food supplement guidelines, along with the whole foods, low fat/salt/sugar, fresh vegetable, and fresh fruit dietary strategy, form the basis for the Cancer Recovery Foundation's approach to nutrition. They are designed to guide and support people in ways to maximize strengthening the body and promoting an optimally functioning immune system.

I recommend that people take vitamin and mineral supplements. Exhaustive and credible research shows that the right levels of nutrients are both protective against developing many cancers as well as supportive of health and healing following a diagnosis.

Ideally we should receive all our nutrients from food. And vitamins cannot take the place of a healthy diet. But even with the best whole food diet, we may have trouble receiving all our required nutrients. Intensive farming practices have led to a demonstrated decline in the nutritional value of certain foods. The result is you may not receive all the nutrients you need in the right amounts all of the time.

In addition, increasing evidence of the negative impact of the wide range of chemicals we are exposed to in everyday life is significant. This calls for an even greater need for nutrients to help with detoxification and protection of the body's organs.

The following guidelines contain information about vitamins, minerals, and other nutritional supplements, along with recommended dosages, that are evidence-based and thought to be specifically supportive for people who have had a cancer diagnosis. Cancer Recovery Foundation developed this program to provide a full range of essential nutrients as well as obtain maximum absorption and bioavailability. For those people who wish to promote their general health and help prevent cancer, these guidelines are also helpful.

Research suggests that vitamins and minerals work best when combined in a way that they all work together, the action of one enhancing the action of others. A high-quality multivitamin and mineral supplement will contain a wide range of vitamins and minerals in levels that allow them to work effectively together. However, if the nutrient levels of your multivitamin are not as high as recommended, I suggest you supplement with individual doses of vitamins and minerals to reach Cancer Recovery Foundation's recommended dosage.

## A Short Overview of Nutritional Supplements and Cancer

All essential nutrients are important for rebuilding and maintaining health. Research shows the following to be particularly beneficial to people with cancer.

### Antioxidants

Antioxidants are the starting point. An antioxidant is a substance that prevents damage caused by excess free radicals in your body. Free radicals are highly reactive chemicals that can damage the DNA in our cells. DNA damage is known to be involved in the development of cancer.

The key antioxidant vitamins are C, E, and beta-carotene (a precursor of vitamin A). They work best in combination. They are especially beneficial in combating the effects of free radical damage to DNA. Selenium is an additional essential mineral that is an important part of antioxidant activity. And coenzyme Q10 is an antioxidant compound made naturally by the body and used by cells to produce controlled cell growth and maintenance. However, when the body's immune function is compromised, the body's natural ability to produce coQ10 is often impaired. These five vitamins and minerals form the basis of the Cancer Recovery Foundation's nutritional supplement program.

A common question is, "Why are the antioxidant doses the Cancer Recovery Foundation suggests higher than the government's recommended daily allowances (RDA)?" The RDA is often set at the level that prevents a deficiency disease, scurvy for example. But this does not necessarily mean that same level will be adequate for supporting maximum health, cancer prevention, or rebuilding the immune system of people with cancer. Cancer Recovery's guidelines meet standards above disease deficiency and therefore must be higher than the RDA.

## Carotenoids

This is a class of natural pigments found principally in plants, algae, and certain bacteria. Carotenoids have antioxidant activity, and some, such as beta-carotene, are converted to vitamin A by the body. Lycopene is a particularly beneficial carotenoid for the prevention and natural treatment of cancer. Fresh organic tomatoes are a rich source of lycopene. In order to maximize absorption, tomatoes are best eaten lightly cooked, then pureed and topped with a splash of extra virgin olive oil.

## Flavonoids

Like carotenoids, flavonoids are one of the groups of plant nutrients with powerful antioxidant characteristics as well as other cancer-fighting properties.

## Omega-3 Fatty Acids

Three fatty acids—ALA (alpha-linolenic acid), DHA (docosahexaenoic acid), and EPA (eicosapentaenoic acid)—are essential to good health. For cancer patients, the fats are particularly important because they support immune function and hormone balance. The best source of the omega-3s is from oily fish, including wild salmon, tuna, mackerel, and sardines. For people unable or choosing not to eat fish, flaxseed (linseed) oil can be a good source. However, flaxseed oil does not contain DHA or EPA. Some brands now add DHA from a plant source.

## Probiotics

Probiotics are supplements of beneficial bacteria that promote gastrointestinal balance. One example is *Lactobacillus acidophilus*. Many cancer treatments are notorious for causing nausea and diarrhea. Most patients can find relief by rebalancing the intestinal tract with probiotics to maintain digestive health. A "detoxified" gastrointestinal track also maximizes the removal of toxins from the body.

### SUPPLEMENTS DURING TREATMENT

Taking supplements during cancer treatment is a subject of intense debate within the cancer community. Cancer Recovery Foundation carefully monitors international research on this subject, constantly updating our recommendations. Following consultation with your oncologist, we currently recommend:

- If you are on a chemotherapy regimen:
  - Continue your multivitamin but suspend your additional supplement program two days (forty-eight hours) prior to receiving treatment.
  - Recommence your additional supplement program three days (seventy-two hours) after receiving treatment.
  - If you are on a continuous infusion treatment protocol, continue your multivitamin but do not take additional supplements during your treatment.
- If you are on a radiation therapy or hormonal therapy regimen, continue to take your multivitamin and additional supplements throughout treatment.

## OTHER NUTRITIONAL SUPPLEMENT ISSUES

Will you still need supplements following treatment? I am a believer. It is the Cancer Recovery Foundation's recommendation that all people with a personal history of cancer take supplements the remainder of their lives. Evidence is clear that proper nutrient levels translate to maximizing health and maintaining healing. In addition, we recommend that people taking supplements over their lifetimes have regular appointments with a nutritional therapist and check our Website, www.cancerrecovery .org, regularly for the most up-to-date nutritional guidelines.

I am frequently asked, "What brand name of supplements are best?" I do not have a good answer. I simply recommend you choose the highest-quality supplements available. The best supplements will contain fewer nonactive ingredients, such as preservatives and binding agents. Higher-quality supplements are also less likely to contain artificial sweeteners and coloring. While this level of supplement tends to be more expensive, I believe the incremental expense to be of value.

Some cancer patients have difficulty swallowing tablets. In fact, "pill burden" is experienced by approximately 25 percent of cancer patients. Simple techniques resolve nearly all these difficulties. Large tablets can be crushed. Capsules can be pierced (please note that lycopene products may stain the teeth). Many vitamins and minerals can be obtained in liquid and powder form. If your concern is complete absorption of the nutrients, choose sublingual products, which are designed to be absorbed under the tongue.

Finally, I would add that you need to keep up to date on nutritional supplement guidelines. Every three months Cancer Recovery Foundation monitors no less than sixteen different sources in twelve countries to review research findings on this important subject. We then review our recommendations and update them when evidence supports such changes.

## CANCER RECOVERY FOUNDATION'S NUTRITIONAL SUPPLEMENTATION GUIDELINES

Supplement Recommendations and Dosages for People with Cancer

*Note: Unless otherwise stated on the label, supplements are best taken with food in order to help maximize absorption.*

**Guidelines for all cancer patients during treatment and thereafter:**

| Nutrient | Details | Daily Dose | Comments |
|----------|---------|------------|----------|
| Multivitamin and mineral | Highest quality affordable | As directed on label | Minimal preservatives, binders, and sweeteners |

**Additional supplements for all cancer patients during treatment, and for two years following treatment, except as noted below:**

| Nutrient | Details | Daily Dose | Comments |
|----------|---------|------------|----------|
| Vitamin B | Part of multivitamin and mineral complex | 50-100mg | |

| Nutrient | Details | Daily Dose | Comments |
|---|---|---|---|
| Vitamin C with flavonoids | Nonacidic ascorbate forms or from foods | 2,000 mg–2g | Take amounts over 1 g in divided doses with meals. |
| Vitamin D | Part of multivitamin and mineral complex | 2,000 mg | Add to multivitamin to reach recommended dosage. |
| Vitamin E | Part of multivitamin and mineral complex | 400 IU | Best taken with vitamin C and beta-carotene. *(Special note on vitamin E: If you have high blood pressure; are taking warfarin, aspirin, or any other antithrombotic drug; are on a chemotherapy regimen; or have a low platelet count, consult your doctor before taking more than 200 IU daily. This vitamin has a mild anticoagulant effect.)* |
| Beta-carotene | Part of multivitamin and mineral complex | 25,000 IU | If you smoke or have smoked in the past ten years, do not take more than 2,000 IU daily. |
| Lycopene | Maximum of 7 mg when taken with beta-carotene | 10–15 mg | Do not take carrot juice at the same time as lycopene. |

| Nutrient | Details | Daily Dose | Comments |
|---|---|---|---|
| Omega-3 fatty acid | Fish oils<br><br>Or . . .<br><br>Flaxseed oil with DHA | EPA + DHA 500 mg or more<br><br><br>1,000 mg | Whole fish oil. No cod oil, which may contain mercury. Vegan alternative for those allergic to fish. |
| Selenium | Part of multivita-min and mineral complex | 200 mcg | |
| Zinc | Part of multivita-min and mineral complex | Women: 20 mg Men: 40 mg | |
| Coenzyme Q10 | Protects heart during chemotherapy | 100 mg | |
| Probiotics | For digestive disorder (nausea, diarrhea) | 1 or 2 capsules, per label | Minimum 1 billion organisms. Keep refrigerated. |
| Milk thistle | For liver health during treatment | 200 mg twice daily | |

## An Important Thing You Can Do

Do your homework. Contact a professional nutritionist. Determine what specific experience he or she has in therapeutic nutritional supplementation for cancer. Compare the nutritionist's recommendations with Cancer Recovery Foundation's recommendations as well as your own research. Be skeptical of unsubstantiated claims. Then, make your own decisions regarding nutritional supplements.

*Important Notice: These statements have not been evaluated by the Food and Drug Administration (FDA). Greg Anderson and Cancer Recovery Foundation make every effort to use up-to-date and reliable sources. However, we cannot accept liability for errors in the sources that we use. Also, we cannot guarantee to provide all the information that may be available concerning your individual health circumstances. All responsibility for interpretation of and action upon the information provided is yours. This information is offered on the understanding that if you intend to support your cancer treatment with complementary or alternative approaches, you will consult with your medical team to be certain they have a complete understanding of your choices.*

# #26

# MAKE
# EXERCISE
# PART OF YOUR
# RECOVERY
# PROGRAM

Hundreds of cancer survivors helped me make an important discovery: Exercise directly correlates with health recovery. Nine out of ten people I interviewed talked about keeping physically active. Even people who were incapacitated or who needed a wheelchair emphasized their commitment to a regular exercise program.

Cancer survivors are markedly different, however, in their exercise goals. Very few set out to run a marathon or become Olympic athletes. Instead, the most common exercise goal among cancer survivors is to experience an increase in energy. In fact, as we previously discussed, moderate exercise, such as a brisk daily walk, is the only known antidote for fatigue.

I chose walking as my exercise. At first I was so weak that even a couple of minutes of walking was too much. So I began with chair exercises, doing simple arm circles—the backstroke movement with my arms fully extended. I'd do ten sets forward and follow with ten sets in the reverse direction. Soon I felt that increase in energy—the deeper breathing, the increase in heart rate, and the better skin color.

It wasn't long before I began to feel stronger. It seemed exercise was working. So I added a few minutes of leg lifts. Soon I was strong enough to put walking back into my exercise routine. Initially, I walked for perhaps five minutes before feeling an increase in energy. But soon that time stretched to ten minutes. Over the months, the exercise periods became longer. I bought an exercise book and added some full-body stretching routines before the start of my walk, and I ended the exercise session with some light calisthenics. I began to feel the combination of physical and emotional regeneration working together to enhance my well-being. You can experience the same.

Today I believe I have found the right balance. Hardly a day passes that I do not walk for at least thirty minutes. I precede the walk with about three minutes of full-body stretches and conclude the session with five minutes of push-ups and sit-ups.

This did not happen overnight. I determined this to be my correct level over a period of two years. Several times I have experimented with exercise beyond the normal thirty-five- to forty-minute daily routine. I tried walking for an hour each day but found I was experiencing hip soreness. I tried weight lifting only to realize I didn't enjoy it.

Some people think more exercise is better. A gentleman recently wrote me to express his opinion that two hours of intense exercise each day is a requirement for cancer recovery. I don't recommend it. Between the threat of injury associated with extended exercise and the rigid, grinding routine that often results in burnout, I believe more harm than good can come from workouts that last two or three hours daily.

Instead, I recommend you find a type of exercise that you enjoy. Then practice that routine just until you feel an increase in energy. The benefits include increased flexibility, greater strength, more cardiovascular capacity, weight loss, and lower blood pressure. But the psychological benefits are even greater—joy, enthusiasm, and mental vitality. What a payoff!

Make exercise part of your cancer recovery program. No matter how long it has been since you have exercised, no matter how incapacitated or confined you are, there are exercises you can do. Exercise will help you get well again.

## An Important Thing You Can Do

Exercise just until you feel an increase in energy. This is your only exercise goal. Do the same tomorrow. Keep extending the duration as you build strength and stamina. No more excuses! Take charge. Your body will respond to this "get-well" signal.

# #27

## GET MORE SLEEP

Fatigue. It's the most common complaint of cancer patients. "I'm always so tired. My radiation treatments drain me," noted Olivia during her recovery from breast cancer. "I just want to sleep all the time. But with all my responsibilities, who has time to sleep?"

Fatigue is part of nearly every cancer patient's experience. Unfortunately, many patients interpret fatigue as an indication of their fast-approaching demise. Not so!

During and just after treatment, you are a different person physically. Just consider what is happening to you. With surgery, a major wound has been inflicted on your body. Chemotherapy puts chemicals into your system that alter your unique biochemical makeup. Radiation causes genetic and cellular changes in your body. Repairs demand rest. No wonder cancer patients are tired.

"For three months I cut back to half days at work," said Ted Chadwick after his bout with bladder cancer. "I took an afternoon nap for a year following my treatment." shared Alicia, who recovered from ovarian cancer. "I still take afternoon naps," said

Bert Byer, celebrating his six-year anniversary of a lung cancer diagnosis.

The fact is, survivors rest. I previously mentioned ginseng as an assist to overcome fatigue. However, no supplement or medication is a replacement for sleep. It is a major mistake to carry on at the same frantic pace to which you were accustomed when you were supposedly healthy. Feeling tired is normal for anyone with any illness. During treatment you may feel tired for weeks until your body gets the opportunity to adjust and recover. So allow yourself rest.

Provided you are getting adequate food and moderate exercise, fatigue is nothing to consume you with worry. It is not a sure sign of your demise. Take that morning nap. Add an afternoon nap if you require it. Or a short rest before dinner may be just what is needed. Eight or more hours of sleep each night is an absolute essential.

## An Important Thing You Can Do

Give yourself permission to get more sleep. Block out rest times on your wellness schedule. Allow your body the rest it needs to repair and heal.

# #28

# FIND A
# POSITIVE
# SUPPORT
# GROUP

**Fact:** Cancer patients who regularly participate in support group meetings live longer than those who do not.

Ongoing research at Stanford University confirmed what cancer survivors have known for decades. In a study of patients with advanced breast cancer, those who attended a weekly two-hour support group session had a life expectancy twice that of the non-attenders. Further research at UCLA and King's College in London confirms the value of attending support groups. The message is clear: We truly need one another for survival.

Distinguish between the two major types of support groups: clinical and psychosocial. The clinical groups communicate basic knowledge on a wide variety of oncology issues. Subjects might include types of cancer treatments, common side effects, physical therapy following breast surgery, or how to live with an ostomy. The idea behind this type of support group is simply to inform.

More critical to survival are the psychosocial support groups. These are the supportive/expressive therapeutic programs that focus on the emotional, psychological, and spiritual aspects of cancer. Look for groups that take a stance of hope without denying the reality of the illness. At meetings you should expect to express your own fears and frustrations freely and allow others in the group to do the same. You'll learn from the responses of the group members who have overcome cancer, and you'll contribute to those who are just beginning the cancer recovery journey.

One warning: A potential problem with any type of support group is that instead of encouraging personal growth, many groups quickly turn into a "pity party." While there is significant value in allowing people to talk out their problems, the discerning group needs a leader to judge when the talking is therapeutic and when it is rehearsing, and reinforcing, a problem. The "cyber-solace" provided in online chat groups is no exception.

When a group of us started Cancer Conquerors support groups, committing to support one another in our wellness quests, we made a pact early on. Each meeting would include a lesson— somebody leading a discussion on a recovery principle—and a time for open discussion and support. The emphasis was to be on the application of lessons that would help contribute to our own healing. It was the smartest move we ever made. We have experienced very few pity parties.

## An Important Thing You Can Do

Contact Cancer Recovery Foundation at www.cancerrecovery.org. A full schedule of our unique Cancer Conqueror Telesupport groups exists. Experience several. Then judge for yourself.

If you don't find what you are looking for, perhaps you need to consider starting a group in your home. Thousands of patients have done so, benefiting themselves and others in their community. Contact Cancer Recovery Foundation of America for start-up information.

# HEAL
# WITH THE
# MIND

Do personal beliefs, positive attitudes, and hopeful expectations make a contribution to cancer recovery? A great deal of credible scientific evidence says "Yes." In fact, the contribution may be greater than science has the ability to measure.

Fighting cancer is much, much more than simply excising a tumor, exposing a malignancy to radiation, or administering chemotherapy through an intravenous drip.

Think bigger. Imagine harnessing all your resources, including the mind/body connection. The basics are actually quite simple. Let's continue our work.

# #29

# STUDY
# THESE
# RESOURCES

Anderson, Greg. *The Cancer Conqueror*. Dallas: Word, 1988. And *Cancer and the Lord's Prayer*. Des Moines: Meredith Books, 2006. Two of my messages of hope and encouragement found through the body-mind-spirit connection.

Benson, Herbert, and Miriam Klipper. *The Relaxation Response*. New York: Quill, 2001. The definitive source for relaxation and meditation concepts and techniques.

Borysenko, Joan. *Minding the Body, Mending the Mind*. New York: Da Capo Lifelong, 2007. How to manage stressful thoughts and uncertainty.

Lerner, Michael. *Choices in Healing: Integrating the Best of Conventional and Complementary Approaches to Cancer*. Cambridge, MA: MIT Press, 1994. The intellectual's guide to alternative treatments.

LeShan, Lawrence. *Cancer as a Turning Point*. New York: Plume, 1994. The emotional aspects of cancer. Helpful exercises involving reflection, discussion, and writing to help come to terms with fears.

Siegel, Bernie. *Love, Medicine & Miracles*. New York: HarperPerennial, 1990. Stories about self-healing from a former surgeon's observations of cancer patients.

Simonton, O. Carl, Stephanie Matthews-Simonton and James Creighton. *Getting Well Again*. Los Angeles: J. P. Tarcher, 1978. Guides cancer patients to participate in recovery through imagery and therapy.

## An Important Thing You Can Do

Visit your bookseller or library. Become immersed in mobilizing your mind for healing.

# #30

## DISCOVER
## YOUR
## BELIEFS

Millions of cancer survivors radically change their beliefs about cancer and about life. Many consider this to be the most fundamental aspect of healing with the mind. I urge you to understand that this idea has a central place in your own recovery efforts.

There are three widely held beliefs that work against overcoming cancer:

1. A diagnosis of cancer means my certain death.
2. The treatment of cancer is drastic, is of questionable effectiveness, and involves many side effects.
3. This diagnosis "just happened" to me, and therefore, there is little I can do to influence it.

All of the above beliefs are untrue! The truth about these statements is:

1. Cancer, no matter how advanced, may or may not mean death.

2. A wide range of treatments do exist and have the potential to be effective. The difficulties in recovery are far outweighed by the benefits.
3. Most illnesses do not "just happen." Our ability to influence health is significant.

These truths can work for you in your recovery. Your response to a problem is more powerful than the problem itself. There is much you can do.

Beliefs have a powerful effect over physical realities. Our beliefs affect the way we perceive illness and literally control our response to it. Beliefs are the determinant of emotions that have a direct link to physical health. In short, our beliefs about ourselves, our disease, our treatment, and our role in healing are inextricably linked with outcomes.

Consciously or unconsciously, our beliefs are creating our reality. It's true both positively and negatively. After interviewing over 16,000 cancer survivors, I know of no survivors who believed that they could not get well. I also have observed that survivors come to understand that beliefs are just thoughts. Thoughts can be changed. If we can bring ourselves to see the central role of beliefs, we can then create self-fulfilling prophecies based on non-limiting beliefs.

Do beliefs affect recovery? Consider this. Beliefs and expectations constantly contribute to actual experiences in all areas of life, including the experience of cancer. If we believe a rainy day means gloom, gloom is what we experience.

I realize it's a long way from rainy days to cancer recovery. But this much is clear: Beliefs can be chosen. The sad fact is we seldom consciously choose them. Perhaps beliefs have simply been accepted by us for many years, like the conventional wisdom surrounding cancer. Perhaps we had beliefs imposed from parents, coworkers, or friends. We may have picked up other people's beliefs and made them our own. They may or may not be true or helpful. But these beliefs have significant power.

Awareness of our fundamental beliefs is often the first, and certainly one of the most dramatic ways to improve our circumstances. If you are harboring the belief that cancer means death, challenge it! The fact is, there are long-term survivors of every type of cancer, including many patients who have been told by doctors that there was no hope.

## An Important Thing You Can Do

Carefully analyze your beliefs. In your Wellness and Recovery Journal, complete the following sentences with the first thought/ feelings that come to mind:

1. One belief I hold about my cancer diagnosis is_____

_____

2. One belief I hold about my cancer treatment is_____

_____

3. One belief I hold about my role in survival is_____

_____

Analyze how your beliefs align with the truths. Talk to others who have successfully traveled the cancer journey. Discover what they believe. Vow to change your self-limiting beliefs today.

# #31

## "REFRAME"
## YOUR CANCER

If you're like most cancer patients, you look upon your illness as the most overwhelming threat to your life you've ever encountered. "I thought of cancer as a powerful evil and deadly force inflicting great injury on me," said Raymond Valrico, a retired restaurant owner who was battling cancer of the larynx. "It was the ultimate threat."

Raymond's words describe his mental outlook. *Cancer . . . a powerful evil and deadly force . . . inflicting great injury . . . the ultimate threat.* It took weeks of counseling, but Raymond came to view his cancer not as a threat but as a *challenge.* Cancer became something that stimulated him to introspection, to review his life. Raymond ultimately made changes in his exercise routine, diet, vocation, and spiritual life. Cancer became Raymond's wake-up call.

Raymond's experience is a perfect example of what it means to reframe the illness. Reframing is the process of finding alternative ways, more positive means, of viewing and responding to any circumstance.

Jose Padilla's diagnosis of prostate cancer was the most frightening and unwelcome event in his fifty-eight years. Even though tests confirmed that the cancer had been discovered early and the prognosis was quite optimistic, his chronic panic-driven thought process focused on his imminent demise. "I don't just have cancer, I was cancer," said Jose.

Frank Cummins also had prostate cancer, but his was significantly more advanced than Jose's. Frank had bone involvement. Unlike Jose, Frank made the critical distinction that he had cancer, the cancer did not have him. "I realized that my mind and spirit had cancer only if I allowed it." Frank's outlook reframed the cancer.

Frank's response demonstrates the significant power we possess. The point of control is not the circumstance of illness; it is our response to the illness. Our response can make all the difference. When we reframe cancer, we respond differently and more proactively. We acknowledge and nourish our inner strength, even in the face of doubt and fear. The threat subsides. We take on the challenge.

Fortunately, both stories have happy endings. Jose was able to embrace many of Frank's more positive beliefs. Today both men are doing well.

## An Important Thing You Can Do

Examine your core beliefs. Then follow this reframing process:

1. What belief about cancer do I want to change?_____

_____

2. What does holding this belief currently gain me?_____

_____

3. How might I come to view cancer as an inspiring challenge rather than a threat?_____

_____

Remember, challenges inspire you to action. Respond to the challenge of cancer.

# #32

# EVALUATE
# YOUR
# SELF-TALK

From the moment we awaken in the morning until we drift off to sleep at night, we experience a constant stream of mental chatter. When we have cancer, our "self-talk" is nearly all negative, filled with fears. It makes for a frightening life experience.

Marion Bricker called Cancer Recovery Foundation in a state of panic, her mind reeling out of control. After the first couple of minutes, I began to jot down the opening phrases of her sentences. They gave a clear picture of her state of mind:

"The cancer is spreading . . ." "I think my insurance is going to be canceled . . ." "How am I going to pay for this?" "It's all such a burden . . ." "I'm afraid of chemotherapy . . ." "My husband can't deal with this . . ." "I feel so frightened . . ." "Why did this happen to me?" "Where is God when you need him?" "There's nothing I can do."

Yes, there is something Marion can do! And you can, too. Believe it or not, we absolutely do choose our every thought. We may think the same fear-filled thought over and over, out of habit, but we are still responsible for that original choice. Analyze the thoughts you have been holding about cancer. That self-talk is the ancestor of your current experience of illness.

Lou Lafferty is a woman who has every excuse needed to lead a life of despair. Childhood abuse, a turbulent early marriage, children in trouble, a toxic divorce, a child who ran away, a second husband who died in a work accident, a serious auto accident after which she was disabled for eight months, and then lymphoma. "My mind," explained Lou, "was always filled with thoughts of life being unfair and difficult, a battle."

Then Lou discovered this great truth: self-talk can change every life experience.

Lou made massive changes. First, she came to the profound realization that her troubles were all in her past, over and done. What happened in the past did not automatically predict what would happen in the future. Of primary importance, Lou came to realize that the thoughts and words she chose right here and now were the ones creating her future. Her self-talk set in place her experience, either good or bad.

That was eight years ago. Today Lou is cancer-free, a happy, healthy, and whole person.

## An Important Thing You Can Do

Complete this awareness-builder. Write down a positive empowering message you can give yourself in the following circumstances.

*Circumstance:* You're frustrated with the doctor for his arrogance, his impatience with your questions, and the limited amount of time he spends with you.

*Positive self-talk:*_____

_____

*Circumstance:* It's 3:00 AM and you're wide awake, consumed with thoughts and fears of suffering and self-pity.

*Positive self-talk:*_____

_____

*Circumstance:* Your energy level is at an all-time low. You are tired and discouraged, questioning if you can take any more.

*Positive self-talk:*_____

_____

Notice what you are thinking at this moment. Is your self-talk negative or positive? Do you wish for your future to be an extension of these thoughts?

# 33

# Choose a Daily Affirmation

Affirmations are positive statements of intent and belief. They take the place of the negative mental chatter that may be gripping you. Affirmations serve to "make firm" the positive things about you and your circumstances. They are consciously chosen self-talk.

Your words are constantly doing one of two things: building you up or tearing you down, healing or destroying. So affirm positively. You are not so much changing the situation as you are changing your thinking about the situation. Changing your thinking about the disease of cancer may be at the heart of experiencing wellness.

Self-talk is the constant conversation of our minds. We process everything, our internal dialogue always interpreting events and creating meaning. Positive affirmations can guide and direct this inner conversation and, in the process, change our response. Affirmations are simply short statements that express the desired outcome. When combined with an acceptance that the old belief is changeable, and the genuine desire to change, we begin to create a new reality.

Affirmations are most powerful when expressed in the present tense. The phrase "I am grateful for life today" is much preferred over a future-tense alternative like "I will show gratitude for my life."

Positive affirmations were first brought to notice in the Western medical world by Emile Coue, a nineteenth-century French pharmacist who noticed that several of his patients dramatically improved when they focused on positive health outcomes rather than the negative fears and images of illness. Coue's famous affirmation, which he encouraged his patients to use, lives on today: *Every day, in every way, I am getting better and better.*

However, affirmations can be exceedingly difficult to believe. It's one of the central reasons that positive thinking is sometimes limited in its effect. An exclusive focus on the positive can result in a sense of unreality. For example, if you have a strong inner belief that you are a bad person and disease is your rightful punishment, telling yourself that you are going to get well is probably not going to work. Predictably, it will be necessary to first recognize the underlying beliefs and challenge the negative ones before the positive ones can be effective.

Affirmation has been dismissed by some people in the medical community as brainwashing. In a way, it is. For years we may have been brainwashing ourselves with limiting beliefs such as, "I am a bad person." When you substitute an opposite and non-limiting belief such as, "I am a child of God, worthy of all God's best," you are deliberately washing your brain with what may seem to be, at first, an artificial construct.

This artificiality is often a problem at first. For example, the affirmation "I am cancer-free" sounds pretty ridiculous when you've just been given the negative results of a CT scan. But the key is to initially pretend, to play with the new belief as if it were true. Our minds cannot yet accept a belief that contradicts the old limits. But it can accept a kind of imagery game in which we play with the new belief as if it were reality. And it is through the play and practice that the new belief gradually becomes believable.

Then we must act. Putting the new desired belief into action confirms and strengthens it. In a spiritual sense, this is acting on faith. You begin to believe that your new belief can be reality and so you act as if it is. At first you do this in very small ways, setting easily attainable goals.

I changed my health with one very powerful affirmation. Right in the middle of the cancer battle, starting at the point where I was down to 112 pounds, confined to bed, and on morphine to control the pain, I began to affirm:

"I am cancer-free, a picture of health. Thank you, God."

I coupled this spoken affirmation with a mental picture of pink healthy cells, a smile on my face, an image of being vital and alive, and my outstretched hands held over my head giving thanks to God. If you came to our home today, you would see a photo of me on a beach, hands lifted overhead, greeting a new day and affirming a new and healthy life.

I would repeat this affirmation countless times—300, 400, even 500 times a day. I'd whisper it. I say it in a normal tone of voice. I'd shout it out loud—at least when no one was at home.

I credit this work of speaking health and healing into my life as the point of power that turned the tide in my cancer journey. Make affirmations work for you. Change your mind and you'll change your health. Whatever we affirm tends to become manifest in our lives. Why not affirm the very best, not out of blindness to illness but out of the well-founded hope of creating your own positive self-fulfilling prophecies of wellness.

Here's how to challenge beliefs and make affirmations work for you:

1. Understand and accept that the old belief is not reality.
2. Nurture a genuine desire to change.
3. Substitute the old belief with the new affirmation.
4. Combine the positive affirmation with positive action.

## An Important Thing You Can Do

Study the following examples. Implement them in your own healing program.

### #1 Limiting Belief

CANCER MEANS DEATH. *Similar beliefs:* Cancer cells are powerful. I am always ill. My body is weak. My resistance is low. I might struggle but the cancer will eventually get me.

### Non-limiting Affirmation

CANCER IS A MESSAGE TO CHANGE. *Similar affirmations:* Cancer cells are weak and confused. I have a healthy body. I am building my immune function. My body has its own inner healing wisdom.

### #2 Limiting Belief

CANCER TREATMENTS ARE TOXIC AND INEFFECTIVE. *Similar beliefs:* I hate my treatments. I always get sick after treatment. I am always so tired after radiation.

### Non-limiting Affirmation

I CHOOSE TREATMENTS THAT HAVE MY "EXCITED" BELIEF. *Similar affirmations:* I believe in my minimally invasive treatment choices. My treatment side effects are readily managed. I am filled with healing energy.

### #3 Limiting Belief

THERE IS NOTHING I CAN DO. *Similar beliefs:* I am a victim of cancer. I have no control over what happens to me. I can't help what I think. I can't help what I feel. I have no choice.

### Non-limiting Affirmation

I AM IN CHARGE OF MY CANCER. *Similar affirmations:* There is a great deal that I can do. I am in charge of my own life. I have many choices. I have great creative resources.

### #4 Limiting Belief

I AM SO AFRAID. *Similar beliefs:* I am helpless. I am trapped. I fear surgery . . . chemotherapy . . . radiation.

### Non-limiting Affirmation

I AM FILLED WITH HOPE. *Similar affirmations:* I am confident. God's spirit of love is within me. I have positive choices.

**#5 Limiting Belief**
I DON'T HAVE ANY ENERGY. *Similar beliefs:* It's too hard for me. I am lazy.
**Non-limiting Affirmation**
I AM ACTIVE. *Similar affirmations:* I have positive energy. Joy and pleasure help me heal.

**#6 Limiting Belief**
IT'S GOING TO TURN OUT BADLY. *Similar beliefs:* I'm unhappy. There's no hope. I don't deserve healing.
**Non-limiting Affirmation**
THIS IS GOING TO TURN OUT PERFECTLY. *Similar affirmations:* I am happy. Life is good. I am worthy of healing. I accept myself as I am now.

**#7 Limiting Belief**
I AM A WEAK PERSON. *Similar beliefs:* I am emotionally . . . intellectually . . . physically . . . spiritually weak. I am not capable of self-healing.
**Non-limiting Affirmation**
I AM STRONG. *Similar affirmations:* I am filled with "heart." I am filled with self-respect. I have a fighting spirit.

**#8 Limiting Belief**
I'M NOT GOOD ENOUGH IN GOD'S EYES. *Similar beliefs:* I'm not worthy. I'm not acceptable to God. I am always wrong . . . guilty . . . inferior . . . a failure. God is out to "get" me.
**Non-limiting Affirmation**
GOD DEEPLY LOVES ME. *Similar affirmations:* I am a good person. God created me. I am a child of God. I accept myself as I am. I respect myself.

**#9 Limiting Belief**
MY DOCTORS DON'T CARE ABOUT ME. *Similar beliefs:* People don't really care. Health-care professionals are only out for

what they can get. My doctor rejects me. My doctor cares only about his/her fee.

**Non-limiting Affirmation**

PEOPLE LIKE AND CARE FOR ME. *Similar affirmations:* My doctor did what he/she did with the best possible motives. He/She really does care for me. I care for myself.

### #10 Limiting Belief

THINGS WILL NEVER GET BETTER. *Similar beliefs:* Things never change. Things are getting worse. I can never change. People in my life can never change. I'll never have the healing I want.

**Non-limiting Affirmation**

EVERY DAY, IN EVERY WAY, I AM GETTING BETTER AND BETTER. *Similar affirmations:* Everything is changing for the better. My healing goes well. I feel good about myself. God is for me. Life is good. This day is good. I am worthy of all God's blessings.

# #34

## MANAGE
## YOUR
## TOXIC
## STRESS

Toxic stress is emotional overload. It is not the circumstances we are experiencing nor is it simply our negative emotions. Toxic stress is the *perception* of overload, the overflow of emotions, sometimes expressed but many times suppressed. This perception is experienced in our minds independent of the circumstances. Importantly, this perception is under our complete control.

Toxic stress only adds to the physical and mental anguish cancer brings. Stress works at cross-purposes to wellness, putting the mind in a state of confusion, blurring the focused peacefulness needed for healing.

There is something you can do about this perception. It's called the "relaxation response." First named and described by Herbert Benson, M.D., a cardiologist and associate professor of medicine at Harvard Medical School, the relaxation response is a simple, effective, self-healing meditation technique for reducing the detrimental effects of all kinds of stress that we live with every day, particularly the stress associated with a life-threatening illness.

Dr. Benson found that the relaxation response is even more

effective when one chooses a focus word or phrase that is closely tied to one's spiritual beliefs. The idea is to pick a word or short passage that has meaning for you: a Christian might use *The Lord is my Shepherd* from the Twenty-third Psalm; a Jewish person might choose *shalom;* a nonreligious phrase might be used, such as the word *peace.*

Pick a phrase with significant personal meaning. Dr. Benson calls this the "faith factor" and explains that it can greatly contribute to helping our minds manage stress more effectively.

The quest for daily self-renewal starts with a decision to handle our problems with a sense of equanimity. Eliciting the relaxation response, especially when coupled with the faith factor, results in our minds working for, rather than against, our wellness.

## An Important Thing You Can Do

Triggering the relaxation response is simple. Try these steps:

1. Find a quiet place, free from distractions, and sit in a comfortable position.
2. Pick a focus word or short phrase that is deeply rooted in your spiritual beliefs.
3. Close your eyes and relax your muscles, from toe to head, particularly relaxing the shoulder and neck area where most tension is carried.
4. Breathe slowly and naturally. Repeat your focus word silently as you exhale.
5. Assume a passive attitude. When a distracting thought comes to mind, simply dismiss it and return to your focus word.
6. Practice this response for ten to twenty minutes twice a day.

In your Wellness and Recovery Journal, check your daily schedule. Do you have time blocked, twice a day, for stress management? Schedule it. Honor these appointments.

# #35

# VISUALIZE
# WELLNESS

An extension of the relaxation process is visualization, also known as mental imagery. This is a valuable tool for helping you reinforce belief in a desired outcome. It is an extension of the relaxation exercises in that it is typically added at or near the end of the meditation period.

The essence of visualization is to 1) create mental pictures of your immune system and of your treatment effectively fighting the cancer. You then 2) visualize the cancer disappearing and your body returning to health. Visualization is that simple, there's no need to make it any more complicated. I urge you to try it.

Consider some of these guidelines: Picture the cancer in symbolic images. For those who require a realistic image, you may want to consult an anatomy text to find pictures of actual cancer cells. Most patients, however, use symbols. I've had people describe their cancer as sand, a lump of clay, and even ice cubes. I saw mine as jelly. The most important criterion for picturing the disease is to think of the cancer as weak and confused. Don't give it power. Your imagery need not be anatomically correct unless you hold a belief that images of correct anatomy are required. What is important is the meaning you give the cancer's imagined symbol; visualize the cancer as weak.

Imagine your treatment as strong and powerful, damaging only the weak cancer cells. Imagine your healthy cells remaining intact. Picture your immune system fighting the cancer. Imagine the weak and damaged cancer cells being naturally flushed out of your body. Picture the cancer shrinking until it is gone. If you are experiencing pain, picture your white blood cells flowing to that area and soothing the pain. Whatever the problem, give your body the command to heal itself, visualizing the process in a way that makes sense to you. End the imagery by seeing yourself well, free of disease, and filled with energy.

How has this benefited you? Most people's fears tend to decrease as the imagery process gives them a greater sense of control. Ongoing research leads us to believe the imagery process has an influence on the body, actually triggering a hormonal and biochemical response to a renewed sense of hope. The resulting changes to the body's chemistry influence immune function, thus assisting the body in maximizing its opportunity to heal.

Visualization is controversial. More than a few health-care professionals consider it to be a form of self-deception. "After all," they reason, "I can show you that the tumor has been growing."

I encourage you to consider this response. In your own mind, separate what is happening from what you wish the outcome to be. It is possible, and beneficial, to picture the cancer shrinking even though it may, at this moment, be growing. This is not self-deception. It is self-direction, and it is necessary to begin the pursuit of any life goal. At first, reality will lag behind the vision you have of the desired outcome. But that vision will tend to pull you in the direction you need to go.

How can you make this technique work for you? After evoking the relaxation response, try this:

1. Picture your cancer cells as weak and confused.
2. Create a mental image of your treatment and your immune system overcoming the cancer.
3. Imagine your body's natural processes eliminating the disease from your system.
4. Envision the cancer shrinking until it disappears.
5. Imagine yourself well, filled with vitality for living.

## An Important Thing You Can Do

Evoke the relaxation response. End it with a visualization exercise. Do so at least twice daily.

# #36

# MINIMIZE TREATMENT SIDE EFFECTS

Conventional wisdom holds that cancer treatments are ineffective and have drastic side effects. Don't believe it. Conventional wisdom needs to be challenged.

Here's the truth: Cancer treatments are becoming more effective every day. Treatments are also becoming more disease-targeted, affecting fewer healthy cells. Plus, several new drugs hold promise for lessening the severity of many of the negative side effects.

Vitally important is the mind's role in combating side effects. In an experiment of a new chemotherapy, part of the group was given saline solution, sterile saltwater, as a placebo. Fully 30 percent of this group lost their hair! It is common for patients to experience nausea, not during or after treatment, but on their way to treatment; this is known as anticipatory nausea. Add to this the legions of examples in which the same treatment results in radically different side effects for different patients, and what do you get? Even allowing for physiological differences, the mind is at work; our beliefs are turned into biological realities.

You and I may perceive our cancer treatments entirely differently. During one of our Cancer Recovery Workshops, I asked Carol, a nursing-home administrator, to draw a picture illustrating her body, her breast cancer, and her treatment.

A few minutes later, she returned with a drawing of a huge devil injecting a charred and smoldering breast with a large syringe of poison. At that same seminar, Rhoda told us that she initially refused both chemotherapy and radiation because she saw them as highly toxic, more threatening than cancer itself. When I asked Rhoda to draw a similar picture, both of her chemotherapy and her radiation therapy, she returned with drawings of chemotherapy as acid eating through a tabletop and radiation therapy as a beam of light that was blinding her vision.

If you believe mind affects body, the implications of these images are significant. Negative perceptions of treatment stand in the way of the body's ability to respond favorably. Whenever a patient sees treatment as a friend, a more positive perception starts to work favorably with the treatment. The best way to make treatment a friend is to make certain you "own" the treatment program, knowing that this is what you consider to be the very best course of action at this time.

The mind is the key. You can program yourself for the most positive outcome possible by using a type of visualization that athletes have successfully employed in training. After evoking the relaxation response, picture yourself sitting in a chair or lying on a table having your treatment administered. In your mind's eye, see the cancer shrinking. Feel your strength returning. At the end of your imaginary treatment, you feel good and ready to enjoy the gifts of renewed health and greater well-being.

If you do this frequently, especially during your course of treatment, evidence suggests your body will respond to the actual treatment with maximum capacity and minimal side effects. Like an Olympic athlete, you will be living the event in your mind first. Your mind helps the body get the message as to how it is expected to respond in the actual situation.

## An Important Thing You Can Do

View your treatment as a friend. Take time, make time, to "imagine" your treatment dramatically helping you. Envision yourself as well, free of any treatment side effects, and returning to radiant health.

The steps in this section are basic and fundamental mind/body principles. There's much more to healing with the mind. You may want to continue your training with more reading, attending seminars and workshops, and perhaps personalized instruction. Start with the source list in section 29. Or contact the Cancer Recovery Foundation at 1-800-238-6479 or www.cancerrecovery.org

# YOUR NEW LIFE
# PERSPECTIVES

It is perhaps difficult to imagine any benefit coming from the experience of cancer. With the frightening diagnosis, the myriad of treatment decisions, and the need to manage all the negative side effects, how could cancer ever be a force for good?

Hundreds of thousands of survivors tell of the real and lasting changes that come directly from their cancer journey. A whole new and better chapter of life has opened before them. I wish this for you, too.

# #37

---

# UNDERSTAND
# THE
# MESSAGE
# OF ILLNESS

When you "reframed" cancer, you began to see illness as more of a challenge than a threat. Now it is time to take this exercise one step further.

The challenge in illness can be found in its message to change. In a real sense, the challenge and message of cancer is a call, an opportunity, for personal growth. In this reframe of cancer lies the seed of true healing and lasting well-being.

Could cancer be a message signaling you to make changes in your life? We've already suggested several changes on the physical level—diet, exercise, and lifestyle issues. Might there be more?

Many survivors view cancer as a call for personal transformation. The changes go beyond physical health habits to changes in attitude and self-image. The wise patient uses the experience of cancer as a turning point, a time to replace ineffective and limited ways of coping by substituting healthier, more effective methods of nurturing relationships, developing vocations, and pursuing spiritual growth.

However, as soon as I suggest this position, people cry, "On some level, you're suggesting I subconsciously gave myself cancer!" Not so! We may have participated, but we did not purposely set out to give ourselves a serious illness. Don't read blame, self-sabotage, or guilt into the message of illness. Instead, realize the changes are potential points of power. Understand that if we have participated in our illness, even subconsciously, then we can participate in our wellness.

Many patients who sincerely explore the message of illness often discover a link between their physical, emotional, and even spiritual states of well-being and the onset of their illness. More important, a large number of the survivors whom I have interviewed can trace the beginning of their healing to their decision to change these beliefs and behaviors. They were able to examine the hidden message in illness and choose a response that changed their lives.

I believe that all of us have a personal responsibility to respond to cancer in this manner. Such a response is in your personal power. Start by asking yourself the following questions:

- *What high-stress events or changes happened in the year or two prior to diagnosis?* Become keenly aware of uncontrollable misfortunes. Death of a spouse or child, loss of a job, and financial setbacks are obvious candidates. Also include internal stresses, such as disappointments, major life adjustments, and ongoing conflict in important personal relationships. Most survivors can identify one or more major stresses in their lives prior to the onset of cancer.

- *What was my emotional response to these circumstances?* Did you process your grief over the loss, express your emotions, and finally adopt a hopeful stance, or did you sink into a chronic depressed state? This is a measure of your participation. Don't read blame here. Participation simply refers to how you responded to the circumstances that may have triggered the stress. Might you have put others' needs before your own? Did you give yourself permission to mourn the loss or did you determine you were going to be invincible and show no emotions? Did you permit yourself to seek the support of others during these stresses? How effective was your emotional self-care? Many survivors gain significant insight from a close examination of these questions.

- *How might my reactions to stress and loss be changed?* Are there alternative ways of responding? Could these toxic circumstances and relationships be removed from your life? If not, how can you balance them, honoring your own emotional needs first?

Give yourself permission to define your true needs. This is highly important wellness work. It is perfectly acceptable to find constructive and uplifting ways to meet these needs, regardless of what others may say or think. Give yourself that permission. Understand the message cancer has for you.

## An Important Thing You Can Do

Conduct a thorough and unflinching personal inventory. In your Wellness and Recovery Journal, complete this exercise:

1. High-stress event(s) that occurred in the year or two prior to diagnosis or recurrence included _____

_____

_____

2. My major emotional responses to these high-stress events were _____

_____

_____

3. I could have changed these circumstances by _____

_____

_____

4.  I could have changed my emotional response by _____

_____

_____

---

*Complete the inventory and then stop your wellness work for today. Carefully contemplate the implications of the important issues raised in this exercise. You may wish to revise your responses after a time of reflection.*

---

# #38

## LIVE
## THIS
## MOMENT

Many people with a diagnosis of cancer needlessly pollute their lives by living in the past or in the future. Instead, I suggest our goal should be to live well with the only time we do have—this very precious present moment.

How many times have you heard yourself say, "If only I hadn't done such and such?" "If only I hadn't smoked." "If only I'd taken better care of myself." "If only . . ." "If only . . ." "If only . . ." We mire ourselves in the regrets of the past and miss the moment we have been given.

At other times we get caught in the fear of the future. "What if the cancer spreads?" "What if the chemo fails?" "What if . . ." "What if . . ." "What if . . ." Here we miss the present moment because we are consumed with what may happen in the future.

The answer: present-moment living. Live now. Live today. Live this hour. All of our regrets about the past, no matter how sincere, won't change history. All our worries about the future won't add even another minute to our lives. On the contrary, both fears and worries diminish our current moments.

Wellness and happiness are not completely dependent on your body's physical condition. High-level wellness is possible even with disability. Appreciate the fact that, even with cancer, you have life, here, now. Living each moment fully is the master secret to well-being.

Wellness has everything to do with the quality of our time; it's about this moment. Don't put off living a full life until you are physically "better." Now is the time! This is your moment!

"I was consumed with worry," said Brenda Barnes, a non-Hodgkin's lymphoma patient, "not just over my cancer, but about my entire life. My parents were divorced and I worried about my mother's emotional health. My dad traveled a lot and I worried about his airplanes crashing. What about my student loans that still hung over my head, unpaid for several years? Why couldn't I maintain a relationship with a man? Was I just an intractable failure in life? And then my illness, on top of it all."

Corwin Johnson was diagnosed with colon cancer at the age of fifty-six. "It (the cancer diagnosis) came two years after my injection molding business failed. All I could think of in those two years was what I should have done differently. If only I had not put so much emphasis on the new product line. Why didn't I see the downturn in the economy? Why did I extend so much credit to our number one customer? I should have announced shorter work weeks or layoffs much sooner. Why didn't I listen to the banker? How am I ever going to get out of debt? If only the family didn't have to suffer. Life is so unfair, I'm ruined."

Brenda and Corwin have a similar problem. Both are absolutely contaminating their present moments. Brenda's worries about the future assure her of enjoying little peace in this moment. Corwin's life is consumed by thoughts of self-judgment that imprison him in the past. Neither is living in the "now." Yet their only chance to capture true wellness is found in the now. What is required is a shift in thinking from what Corwin might have done in the past or what may happen to Brenda in the future, to what each can do right here, right now. What about you? Might similar shifts be required?

Our potential for knowing wellness depends on our ability to understand that the past does not equal the future. Living in the now frees us from an internal bondage that keeps us from following the wellness path.

The past is over. Regrets, remorse, and recrimination cannot touch us unless we allow them to remain in our lives. The future cannot harm us unless we create a future based on perceptions of fear, anger, and guilt. The only time that contains the power to change our lives is the present moment.

Just because you have cancer now does not predict, with certainty, that you will have it next year. Understand that truth. You have power in this moment that can change your life. Exercise that power—now!

## An Important Thing You Can Do

Each day, relinquish any thoughts or judgments that hold you to the past. Give up any fears that keep you from creating a healthy future. Pick one activity this day, this moment, that brings you pleasure, contentment, and happiness. Do it now! Know that the supply of these moments is limitless, there for the taking if you will only choose to do so. Here, in the present moment, you will find your wellness.

# #39

# Take Time to Play

How much time have you allowed yourself for play in the last week? If you answered "None," you are a member of a very large club. That's unfortunate. Living well requires play.

It's a common phenomenon. Many adults react negatively to the idea that we need to play. In fact, millions of people believe that grown-ups should not play. Somehow we think that playing is not the mature thing to do. Challenge this thinking. From this moment forward, I want you to understand that play is an important part of your "work" of wellness!

The need to honor our playful nature is very strong. Most of us just repress it. Don't. Give yourself permission to play, actually scheduling play time in your daily calendar if you must. I did. We must then treat that time carefully, assigning it the same importance and priority as other areas of life, such as work and family.

Sometimes we get fooled into thinking we are playing when we really are not. Eli Goldman, who was diagnosed with multiple myeloma, was also a member of a barbershop quartet. He thought his singing was play. Then Eli began to look at his "play" more closely. He soon realized his singing wasn't as much play as it was competition, a pressure to win contests, a pressure he did not need. Eli dropped out of the quartet and substituted kite making, in which the competition was strictly self-imposed. What a valuable lesson!

Analyze your own life. Have you noticed that you're never too tired to play? In fact, if you think you're tired, perhaps that is just the signal that you need more play. Play builds energy reserves; it is a major contributor to wellness.

God didn't create us just to work, work, and work. We were created for joy. So create some joy in your life. Consider this list of ten noncompetitive play activities:

1. Stroll on the beach.
2. Fly a kite.
3. Swim.
4. Ride a bike.
5. Draw a picture.
6. Write a poem.
7. Skip around the yard.
8. Sing.
9. Listen to music.
10. Take the scenic route.

## An Important Thing You Can Do

Make your own play list and record it in your Wellness and Recovery Journal. Now, I want you to stop reading. Put aside this book, right now, and go play for thirty minutes. Go! Have some fun. Do it! We'll continue our wellness work later.

# #40

# LAUGH FOR HEALING POWER

Norman Cousins made many contributions to our understanding of the mind's role in mobilizing the body's healing processes. But none is so vividly remembered as his emphasis on laughter. In his 1981 book, *Anatomy of an Illness*, Cousins called laughter "internal jogging." Since that time, science has confirmed that even something as simple as a laugh or a smile carries with it a positive biochemical response.

The message is clear: Lighten up! It will directly enhance your well-being. Just notice how relaxed you feel after laughing at a good story or watching a funny movie. It's wonderful!

Jack Abrams is a New York investment banker, successful, wealthy, the owner of a beautiful home in Westchester County, and the recipient of a metastatic prostate cancer diagnosis. "I thought, my God, I'm going to die. Cancer was the most god-awful threat I had ever faced." Jack received radiation treatment at a Manhattan medical center where he met Delmar, an older gentleman who always had a humorous story to share. Delmar had successfully completed the same treatment for prostate cancer some seven years earlier. Now he volunteers three days a week at the hospital. "My job," said Delmar, "is court jester!"

For most of us, seriousness is seen as an important virtue. "Gravitas" we call it. We tend to think that laughing or giggling is childish behavior and certainly not appropriate for adults. Jack used to subscribe to this thinking. "After all," he remarked, "investment banking is serious business. You have to be serious to be taken seriously."

Baloney! I observe way too many cancer patients going through life with this fearful, beaten, and downtrodden seriousness surrounding them. There is nothing inconsistent about being an adult and including laughter in your life. There is nothing wrong with being ill and pursuing a lighthearted approach to wellness. This is not some demented form of personal denial. Instead, it can be the opportunity to let the hidden child in you come out once in a while. Get in touch with that exuberant, vibrant part of yourself. Enjoy playing with your own children or grandchildren. Laugh at yourself and your seriousness.

Jack reflected, "Delmar taught me a lot about living. When I stopped being so serious, I started to get well."

## An Important Thing You Can Do

Go ahead. Rent that comedy DVD. Watch your favorite sitcom. Go to the local comedy club or a silly movie. Laugh! Let those positive biochemicals loose. It's healing.

# #41

# EVALUATE
# YOUR
# RELATIONSHIPS

Our relationships. We constantly interact with other people—a husband or wife, a friend or a lover, a child or a relative, a boss, a coworker, or an employee; the list of our relationships is endless. At times, our lives seem to center entirely on relationships. How we get along with the significant people in our lives seems to determine, to a large extent, the quality of life we have. Furthermore, the absence of relationships can cause much disharmony and deep dissatisfaction. Like it or not, relationships are central to our experience of life and even our experience of illness.

Cancer survivors invest time and energy in two-way relationships that nurture them. Survivors put relationships that are toxic "on hold." Patricia shared in a support group meeting what this meant to her. "I had to move out. It was difficult, particularly leaving my two children. But I knew it was what I needed at that time. And I stayed away for nearly three months."

Patricia married while in college. She went to work to support her husband and his education. Patricia was expecting her first child before her husband graduated from dental school. She never earned her degree, something her husband seemed to hold over her.

"He was always criticizing me," Patricia said. "And I would yell back, trying to defend myself from attack. I'd bring up times when he disappointed me. And he would counter with a litany of my shortcomings. It became a vicious cycle. So I got out of there."

Was a marriage gone askew partly responsible for Patricia's cervical cancer? I believe so. Toxic stress lowers our resistance. Sadly, Patricia's search for love led to an extramarital affair. The guilt became overwhelming, leading to clinical depression. Patricia came to believe the breach in her marriage was linked to her physical problems. After beginning her cancer treatment program, she finally began to look at the relationship with her husband.

Credit Patricia with wanting the relationship to work. With the help of a marriage counselor she was able to better understand her part in the ongoing battles. Patricia recognized her reactions and began to select other more measured responses to her husband's remarks. Today, Patricia and her husband are working on improving their relationship, and Patricia is cancer-free.

Here's a key insight you can use to your tremendous benefit. Our relationships with others often reflect the relationship we have with ourselves. Do you experience conflict with a coworker? Look within to understand the inner conflict you may carry. Does a child seem self-willed and impossible? Look within. Do you carry a belief that kids are willful and impossible?

Your self-perceptions are exceedingly powerful. They dramatically impact our relationships. And spiritually, even though we may have some changes of perception to make, it's the set of the heart that matters. If our hearts are in the right place—on the path of love, joy, and peace—our spiritual well-being is assured. All this takes is an internal search of our motives.

This internal search is our only real point of influence. When we evaluate relationships, the central task is to look within, discovering the truth: The only way to change another is to change ourselves first.

Be an encourager in all your relationships. Know that whatever you send out will always come back to you. Change and improve your relationships by sending out the love, joy, and peace that will help you heal. Truly, this is your point of power.

Do healed relationships always equate with healed bodies? I believe the two go together, but I can cite only anecdotal evidence. When we stop punishing ourselves and others for things that happened in the past, we are then free to move on to a life of wellness, at state of mind and spirit that often supports vast and rapid physical improvement.

## An Important Thing You Can Do

Conduct an inventory of the ten most important relationships in your life. Number a page in your Wellness and Recovery Journal from 1 through 10 and record the people's names. Did you realize these were the ten most important people in your life?

Highlight any relationships that need to be put on hold. Are there any that need improvement? Indicate those. What is one thing you could change that would improve each relationship?

Come back to this list often. Keep it current. Declare any "relationship war" to be over! Declare that you now live in joy and peace. Appreciate how important this work is to your achievement of wellness.

# #42

# GET
# BEYOND
# "WHY?"

It's the inevitable question cancer patients ask: "Why did this happen to me?"

The trouble with the "why?" question is that we seldom like the answers we are given. We fight them, not wanting to accept. Some think cancer is a lifestyle issue: "He smoked." That may be true for some but does not stand up to scrutiny for all cancer patients or even all smokers. Others say the "why?" is environmental: "We've polluted the planet. We're all getting sick." That may explain some cases, but why is it that other people exposed to the same carcinogens remain perfectly healthy?

Religion tries to answer the "Why me?" question. I've been told by well-meaning clergy that God was using cancer to punish my sins, to correct me for my eternal profit, to draw me closer to God, and to help me and my family members learn submission. Incredible!

When we ask "why?" we are often looking for someone or something to blame. "Why?" is another way of saying we are helpless and the situation is beyond our control. Some people blame others, some blame circumstances, some blame parents, some blame doctors, some blame the environment, and some blame God. Affixing blame does not help. It only creates helpless victims, something I trust by now you believe you are not.

The road to personal wellness starts when we stop asking "why?" and begin to consider the question, "Toward what end?" or "For what purpose?" Put another way, "How can I make this experience benefit myself, others, and the world?"

Literally thousands of the cancer survivors I have interviewed and surveyed speak of "God not being done with me quite yet." Could that be the case with you? Instead of asking, "Why me?" let's ask, "Heavenly Father, what more can I do to serve you?" Then quiet yourself and listen. Let this idea settle deep in your spirit. It's the essence of getting beyond the "why?" of cancer.

## An Important Thing You Can Do

In your Wellness and Recovery Journal, start a new page with the heading "How can I make my experience of cancer beneficial?" Describe, in writing, how you believe cancer can help you and others. Continually add to this list as your insights deepen.

# #43

# PRACTICE
# SELF-DISCIPLINE

Living a life based on maximizing your well-being requires living with values and behaviors that may be radically different from the ones you had before your illness. Some days, the work of wellness may not be the easiest or most convenient to practice. On a cold and rainy morning, it might be easier to stay in bed and forget the exercise. And instead of preparing a high-nutrition lunch, it might seem simpler to use the drive-through window of the nearest fast-food restaurant. Our intention to move toward wellness may seem strong, but too often our practices may not reflect that intent.

I encourage you to see yourself as self-disciplined. Wellness self-discipline includes thought and deed, intent and practice. This principle is equally valid whether you are facing a just-baked batch of chocolate-chip cookies, a dark cold morning of exercise, or an unforgivable person. Gentle, wholesome self-discipline is at the core of making wellness real in your life.

The issue is not whether we *can* choose wellness. It's whether we *see ourselves* choosing wellness. Remember Robert Schuller's encouragement, "The me I see is the me I'll be."

The practice of seeing yourself as self-disciplined leads to two very powerful life qualities: self-respect and freedom. When your walk matches your talk, when intent and action are one, you have a consistency in your life that is unshakable. You are grounded in a principle-oriented life experience, firm in the knowledge that all you are doing physically, emotionally, and spiritually is in your best interest.

Just for a moment, envision yourself as happily self-disciplined. Inner strength and self-respect flow from this position. The discipline to actually act on what is important to you leads to personal freedom; you are no longer bound by the traps of obsession, compulsion, and self-pity. This is a personal power at the highest level, a strong and quiet inner assurance that is one of the rewards of the wellness journey.

When I get up in the morning, the first thing I do is pull on my sweats and running shoes. No excuses. I discipline myself to exercise.

Diet was a wellness discipline that challenged me. I loved sweets, especially pastries. Today, I simply do not allow myself to indulge. I deserve better nutrition. Discipline.

Meditation—when do I have time to fit this into a busy schedule? Yet I do, twice each day. Dicipline. My times of meditation result in a clearer perspective on the day, a perspective that I refuse to live without.

The same is true for developing a purpose/play balance, nurturing my relationships, and honoring my spiritual needs. Each important area of my life requires a consistent disciplined practice in order for me to know its potential. I see you doing something very similar. It starts with seeing yourself as self-disciplined and actually doing the work of wellness.

"But that's no fun," protested Manuel Morales, a big, burly mechanical engineer with kidney cancer. He was attending one of our workshops in San Antonio. "You're right," I responded, "It's better than fun. It's freedom—freedom from all that hurts us."

Self-discipline. The issue becomes which habits we will

choose in our lives. Choose a positive addiction. Decide to discipline yourself to choose the habits of wellness. The result is self-respect and freedom.

## An Important Thing You Can Do

Match your walk with your talk, your actions with your best intentions. Pick one area—perhaps diet or exercise—and make that your focus today. For example, pick one day and excel at maximizing your nutrition. Then choose another area for focus for the next day. And another the next. Feel your self-respect skyrocket. Congratulate yourself. Bask in the personal power and freedom this discipline brings to you.

# #44

## CHOOSE YOUR EMOTIONAL STYLE

What is your dominant style of expressing emotion? Is it suppression, where you constantly restrain yourself from venting real feelings; or overreaction, where you are too exuberant or fly into inappropriate rage; or denial, where you tend to push feelings out of your consciousness?

If you have read this book to this point, you now know that emotions have a central role in wellness. Two emotional styles concern me most: fear that is denied and hostility that is either suppressed or overexpressed. Our goal here is to become a skilled observer of our emotional reactions and learn the ability to choose appropriate responses.

You have the right to feel any emotion. Any and every emotion you feel is perfectly acceptable. We're human; we feel. In a real sense, we are emotionally driven creatures. One moment we're angry, the next moment we're down. We're happy and we laugh. The next moment we're fearful of some loss. I've observed that people tend to repeatedly experience four basic emotions: mad, sad, glad, and e'gad—anger, depression, happiness, and fear. All of them are acceptable.

To experience an emotion, and recognize that any emotion is acceptable, is one level of understanding. But the healthful processing of those emotions is quite another. It's here we typically find trouble.

You have tremendous power over your emotions. It's the power of choice. Health-enhancing emotional processing is summarized by the phrase *review, release, and renew.*

Review the emotion. The most damaging mistake we make in emotional expression is to attach too high a priority on either burying or venting the feeling. Instead, start by observing the emotion. Review it. Understand it. That's half the challenge.

Then release the emotion. Get rid of the anger, the sadness, the fear. It's perfectly acceptable to feel the way you feel. It's your emotion and you own it. But then release it in a nonhostile way, without being coy, subtle, or vague. Think or say, "I'm upset but it's only my emotions. It's over and done. Life goes on." Release.

Then renew. Think and say, "I can choose my emotions. My emotions do not choose me." You replace it. Consciously, cognitively, you choose a more productive, more loving, more spiritual emotional response.

This process is so very powerful. For example, my personal emotional challenge is effectively processing anger, one of the most highly charged emotions. My anger is generally short-lived, a negative emotion over a single event. When I'm functioning at my best, I'll review it: "There's my anger. I recognize it. It's starting to boil my water." Then I'll release it: "Anger. Go away. I become upset when you're around." I express it, without malice. I release it.

The trouble comes when I don't renew, when I fail to consciously replace that anger with love, or at least compassion. When I allow anger to continue to control my responses, I am plagued by chronic anger that wears a mask. It appears to be anger but it is actually unresolved hostility—toxic emotions and feelings to which I cling. It's like walking through a field that is filled with landmines. The slightest nudge and an explosion erupts.

One of the demands of living well is to no longer cling to negative emotions. We cling with coping styles of denial, suppression, and overreaction. Not until we review, release, and honestly renew can we become masters of our emotions.

You also have this power. Renewal is actually very simple. For me it comes when I focus my attention on what actually provoked me. If I will just reflect on the event, I will often discover that I perceived the provoker—be it a person, event, or condition— with fear. I was the one who was fearful that my person, property, or pride was under attack.

This is a profound discovery of the highest importance, one that affects us on every level of our lives. It's fear we are dealing with, actually our perception of fear, something that is under our control. Now we can review and release that fear, and verbalize it. "This diagnosis scares me." Or, "Doctor, I reject that prognosis."

Then, and only then, can we transcend emotionally. We renew; we consciously choose a more powerful and productive emotion. "I choose to be hopeful—anyway."

That's why it is so important that we become keenly aware of our emotional style. Simply observing the situations that trigger our emotions allows us to rethink our perception that we are under siege. Instead of perceiving fear, we can now understand the situation in the light of love, or at least compassion. This is a new and miraculous emotional response, one that immediately begins to dissolve resentments and helps immensely in our healing.

Make it your priority to become a keen observer of your own emotions. Review, release, and renew. It is the secret to emotional well-being.

## An Important Thing You Can Do

Become an objective observer over the next week. When an upsetting event occurs, record the event in your Wellness and Recovery Journal. Then record your emotional response based on one of three categories: denial—"I denied that there was any problem"; suppression—"I suppressed my emotions when I really wanted to tell them off"; or overreaction—"I went crazy and overreacted, way out of proportion to the whole event."

Then practice the three Rs: review, release, and renew. You'll become a skilled observer of your own emotional stance toward life. Reactions and emotions that were once automatic will now come under your control. Through it all, you will achieve new levels of well-being.

# FOR THE COMMITTED

I trust you have been following and implementing the steps in this book. If so, you are well on your way to triumph over cancer.

Many cancer survivors go even further, reaching for higher levels of well-being in all areas of their lives.

"I see it [cancer] as a gift," said singer Olivia Newton-John about her journey through breast cancer. "I know it sounds strange. But I don't think I would have grown in the areas I did without this experience."

Seek the gift in cancer. It's there. Join me now in continuing this search.

# #45

# SEE
# LIFE
# THROUGH
# SPIRITUAL
# EYES

What do you see when you look at your life? Do you see a body riddled with disease, dreams shopelessly derailed, a family frightened and life lived in despair?

Or can you see a precious moment, a special instant in space and time where mind and spirit are ill only if you allow it? Can you see the beauty and grace, even the perfection, in your life without coloring those qualities with the pain of cancer?

Peter Halters was a forty-year-old father who developed pancreatic cancer. It was a difficult battle, especially since he wanted so very much to live. His valiant efforts were an inspiration to many people. During one of our telephone sessions, Peter remarked, "I think the spiritual part began to make sense last night. We were at the dinner table, the whole family. And I saw something different. It really stuck with me."

"What do you mean?" I asked.

"Well, before last night, I always saw the obvious at the dinner table: the chicken, the salad, and the mashed potatoes. I'd see my wife, looking tired and worried like she was always running behind schedule. And the kids with a thousand stories of things happening at school. That was what was in front of me. That's what I saw.

"But last night I saw from my heart," continued Peter, struggling to hold back tears. "I looked around that table and saw something quite different. For the first time, I was able to see this precious moment where the minds, bodies, and souls of our family were gathered together to break bread and be nourished. There was so much more there than just the food. There were lives filled with potential for good. We were there to help each other, to love and care for each other."

Peter paused as he relived that special moment in his mind. "Then the children got into an argument with their mother. But instead of driving me up the wall, this conflict was somehow different. Or at least I saw it differently. It seemed to be a natural expression of love toward each other, a way of saying, 'I care.'"

Peter was looking through spiritual eyes. Spiritual eyes allow us to see the value of what is simple and readily available in our lives in spite of the circumstances in which we may find ourselves.

"I awoke from my surgery," said Pontea Kamal, "and there in my room was my husband. He was holding our little daughter, propping her up on the hospital bed. And she was squeezing my finger. Her big dark eyes looked at me, and she smiled as she said, 'I love you, Mommy.' It was such a precious moment. Now, since my cancer, I see so much deeper into life."

Make a commitment. Join me in no longer dwelling on what is wrong and taking inventory of what is missing. Let's put our focus on all that is right, all that we have. And we have a lot.

This level of awareness brings a vastly different experience of cancer and of life. Embrace this consciousness. There are miraculous moments in your life right now—each and every day. See them.

## An Important Thing You Can Do

Stop. Take a few minutes to see life in this new, more spiritual light. Ask yourself, "What do my countless blessings really mean to me?" This new awareness may contribute more toward your well-being than the most potent medicine.

# #46

# VALUE PERSONAL SPIRITUAL GROWTH

Too many people equate victory over cancer with a doctor's report that says, "This patient is clinically free of cancer." I understand that desire, I share that desire, and, in fact, my records state exactly that. I wish you the same. But that is not the most important part of the journey through cancer.

Please read carefully. Consider these next words deeply. For the person who opens his or her mind and spirit, the cancer experience evolves into a transcendent spiritual journey. The real triumph over cancer is realized in the nurturing of personal spiritual growth.

Some people say, "Greg, I'll settle for a cure. Just get my life back to normal." Don't settle for that! You don't want things to get back to normal. After your experience with cancer, things will never be the same again. You want a new and better life. That life comes in the form of a new spiritual walk.

Cancer has pounded you with a million hammer blows. But you have the last word as to how those blows will shape you. William James, the distinguished psychologist and philosopher, declared that his generation's most important discovery was that human beings, by changing their inner attitudes of mind, could change the outer aspects of their lives.

I see you changing in that way, using the hammer blows of cancer to change your inner state of spirit. By making personal spiritual growth our aim, the most important discovery will be to use the experience of cancer to shape us into wonderfully different people. Indeed, cancer can reshape our attitudes, soften our spirits, and transform our lives.

It's personal spiritual growth we seek. You have those seeds of well-being inside you. But it's up to you to believe and act on them.

Think of personal spiritual growth as the natural and logical extension of your wellness journey. The steps are simple. You are going to make a decision to do all possible to get well again. You are going to devote time and energy to understanding your treatment options, to improving your diet, to daily exercise, to making positive beliefs and attitudes real in your life, and to nurturing your most important relationships.

Then, in a very seamless progression, you'll explore and develop your own practices of gratitude, forgiveness, unconditional love, and more. It's the spiritual part of the wellness journey.

Are you ready? It's the most important part of the trip.

Cynicism has no place here. You cannot climb up the spiritual mountain by thinking downhill thoughts. If you feel that life is filled with despair, that it is gloomy and hopeless, and that spiritual growth is impossible for you, it is because you are gloomy and hopeless. You must change your inner world, which will in turn change your outer world.

Powerful healing awaits you. Associate with people who are walking the spiritual path. Your spiritual journey can be advanced by meeting and mingling with those who have a spiritual vision. Be inspired by our great spiritual ancestors from all the ages.

And pray. Be still and prayerfully listen to God. Don't beg or plead. Pray, "Thy will be done." Then listen. And then act.

Please, don't limit God's infinite possibilities by imposing your conditions for wellness. God can use you even with cancer. Be open to that spiritual experience. Remember, with God, all things are possible.

## An Important Thing You Can Do

In your Wellness and Recovery Journal, record one spiritual quality that you would like to make vivid and real in your life. Start by making a commitment to practice that quality for just one hour. Then extend the time. Keep this as your central goal. Pray and listen for guidance. Opportunities for practice will present themselves every moment of the day. Seize them.

# #47

---

# MAKE
# FORGIVENESS
# A HABIT

Do you want to free all your energy to heal? Forgive! Let go!
Release!

Forgiveness is wellness work that brings with it huge rewards.
Forgiveness links our newfound awareness of the healing dynam-
ics with our awakened understanding of our emotional style. The
promised benefit of this linkage is the emotional and spiritual
peace and serenity we need for healing.

This is a big promise. Forgiveness can deliver.

I believe forgiveness, when it actually becomes a way of
thinking and living, is the single most powerful key to wellness.
Forgiveness is a trusted technique by which our thoughts and
perceptions are changed, transforming the harmful effects of toxic
emotions into the healing reality of compassion, even love. Forgiveness allows us to switch our focus from fear to love; it helps
us change what can be changed and allows us to make peace with
the rest—a profound dimension of healing.

Opportunities to learn and practice forgiveness are everywhere.
The obvious teachers of forgiveness come in the form of people,

most often individuals who antagonize us, the ones whom we can't stand to be around.

But more important than forgiving others is teaching ourselves to be self-forgiving. It all starts with our own power and control.

Let's be honest; we hold much resentment and shame against ourselves; we don't let go easily. In the quiet moments we judge ourselves harshly: "I'm so stupid. I'm fat. I'm ugly. I'm not worthy. I probably deserve this illness." The list is without end.

Now, with cancer, like never before, this is the moment to release that self-condemnation. The only way is through self-forgiveness.

Let go. I observe so many cancer patients carrying self-concepts of unworthiness. These are false and deadly beliefs. Yes, we may have done something undesirable, but that is our behavior and does not equate with being an unworthy person. Release those feelings of unworthiness.

A young single mother shared, "I was a drug addict and a prostitute. Now cancer. But I think I deserve it. God is punishing me."

"No," I responded. "Absolutely not! Release those beliefs. They are serving only to condemn you to a life of disease. Forgive yourself. Forgive others. Ask God to forgive you. Release it all."

There's more. Beyond ourselves, our perceptions of others can also create a battleground of emotional turmoil. It is so easy to judge others. Judgmental behavior tears at the fabric of relationships and kindles the fires of resentment. Cancer is, among other things, an opportunity to learn and practice the difference between acceptance and approval, to transcend judgment.

I urge you to practice acceptance. A man with metastatic prostate cancer came to our offices and soon began to tell the tale of his son who was gay. There was so much strife between the two—fights, accusations, condemnation. The son left for college and never returned home. For over six years, the two hardly spoke. It weighed so heavily on the father. Then he got his cancer diagnosis.

"I knew that forgiveness and reconciliation were central to my getting well again," said the man. "I finally reached my son on the phone and said I would like to see him. When we met, the first thing I promised was to never again mention his lifestyle. I made a decision to release it all—his lifestyle and my health—to God."

Forgive. Let go. Release. Yes, forgiveness is *the* answer. All of us have imperfect natures. All of us exhibit behaviors that don't match our potential. Forgiveness allows us to accept imperfection without having to approve of it. Have you noticed? Not everything in life meets your expectations. But we can find peace through acceptance. Yes, we still distinguish right from wrong. But forgiving ourselves and others is at the heart of practicing acceptance. Let go.

Join me. Let's begin to make the practice of forgiveness a habit. Forgiveness is experienced on two levels. The first is the most obvious. There is an event: Someone is wronged or we perceive an attack. That behavior needs to be forgiven. When we can say, "I forgive myself for _____," or "I forgive _____ (another) for _____," then we have embarked upon the forgiveness journey.

The second level of forgiveness changes our perception of what happened. Yes, an event occurred. But the real problem starts when we begin to judge what happened, when we label ourselves or the other person as bad, hurtful, mean, stupid, or with some other less-than-kind attribute. We perceived the event as unfavorable; the event didn't meet our approval. We judge, even condemn, the people involved.

The alternative? Acceptance. Accept ourselves. Accept others. Accept that events happen. Accept that life is often far from our glittering ideals. Forgive and accept. This is a far better way to live.

People who are, or believe themselves to be near death often come to the realization that forgiveness heals. Feuds, differences, and deep hurts suddenly seem less important at this time. I can understand. I had to learn this lesson myself. Literally thousands of patients share similar stories.

Marilyn Ellis, in the middle of a battle with ovarian cancer, felt terribly ill at ease when her mother and father visited. Marilyn and her mother would make noble efforts to get along with each other, but they seldom fully succeeded. Old patterns of attack and defense were constantly cropping up between them. Child care, cooking, homemaking, religion—the particulars didn't seem to matter. Her mother wanted a more conservative daughter. Marilyn wanted a more enlightened mother.

"It was driving me crazy," said Marilyn. "During her last visit, I was ready to throw her out. But then it occurred to me, God isn't looking at my mother and thinking, 'Mildred is so impossible.' How could I pretend to want to get along with my mother if I was so consumed by my judgment of her errors? I had to practice acceptance and get off my fixation with approval.

"So I said to myself, 'I'll try this for an afternoon. I'll focus on acceptance and give up approval.' From that moment, the situation and the relationship started to shift. As I was more accepting of her, she became more accepting of me. We're a long way from best buddies," conceded Marilyn, "but there is a growing bond between us."

Maybe you struggle with hostility and resentment. If so, forgive. The amazing payoff of forgiveness is that so many people do get well after letting go. Lives are certainly made better; many are made longer. But it strikes me that if one is willing to forgive during the last moments of life, why not do it earlier? Like right now?

How often do we need to forgive? Always. Don't drag the memories of past hurts and mistakes into your present moments. Nothing from the past is important enough to allow it to pollute our present. Forgive. Let go of judgment. Become a shining example of compassion. You deserve it. You'll change your life—forever!

## An Important Thing You Can Do

Choose just one hurt or mistake and forgive everyone concerned with it. Say out loud, "(Name), I totally and completely forgive you. I release you to the care of God. I affirm your highest good." Mean it. Now feel the warmth of forgiveness. Choose to forgive one person each day.

# #48

---

# EXUDE
# GRATITUDE

What is the least-healthy spiritual habit, the one that causes disease of every kind? It's ingratitude—the lack of thankfulness, our inadequate appreciation for all the blessings we enjoy.

Have you expressed your thankfulness today? We all have so many blessings to appreciate every day of our lives. But most of us overlook them. The conscious practice of being grateful is central to the healing process.

Even with cancer, even in the middle of a difficult treatment cycle, even in your darkest and most fearful hours, be thankful for all you do have. For life, for love, for family, for friends, for the awesome beauty of nature, for the presence of God, for all these things and more, be thankful.

Why do I feel so strongly about gratitude's healing power? It's because I have seen gratitude bring more significant and rapid improvements to the lives of cancer patients than any other single action. Thousands of survivors are convinced that there is a physiological correlative to gratitude, and their bodies respond. I agree.

Be grateful. If you wish to cultivate a deeper attitude of gratitude, I suggest you begin to see yourself as a guest who is only
visiting here on earth. All that you have is not really yours; it is a
gracious gift from your host. You are privileged to enjoy the gifts
of friends and family, home and transportation, food and recre-
ation, vocation and service, during your stay. Even your health,
no matter what the state, is another of those gifts.

Jill Phillips lay near death in a small rural Nebraska hospital
after being told she was "filled" with cancer and that it was inoperable. Mired in despair and self-pity, she could see nothing for
which she could be thankful. "I was divorced, my two children
were grown and lived in different parts of the country. I hated my
dead-end job. My life seemed miserable.

"But one night I looked out of my hospital window to see a
deep, dark sky that was filled with stars. I shut off all the lights
in my room and just gazed at the sky for what must have been
hours. I started to ask a lot of questions: 'What is this huge uni-
verse about? What is my place in it? Why am I sick?' I can't say I
got a lot of answers. But I did get a different perspective.

"I became thankful," continued Jill, "grateful just for being a
part of this huge and wonderful world. I realized that in my fifty-
plus years, I had been able to experience so much. The marvel
of giving birth to two other lives—what a miracle! The beauty of
the country, where I feel such strong roots; I was so grateful to
live here rather than in a city. The deep friendship I had with my
sister—I was so thankful for her love. That night at the window
changed my whole perspective on my problems."

Like Jill, we too can capture true well-being when we choose
gratitude. But so many roadblocks on the cancer journey seem to
detour us, to mire us in ruts of ingratitude and self-pity. We're so
busy with appointments and treatments, discomfort and despair,
fear and pain, that we lose our perspective. We tend to look at the
cancer journey as a long and twisted path, filled with potholes.
There seems to be nothing for which we can be thankful. This is
faulty and self-destructive thinking.

Every day start saying aloud, "I am so grateful for all I have been given, even my next breath." Exude gratitude. It transforms the very experience of illness and of life. I implore you, see beyond the day-to-day experiences that seem so all-consuming. Treasure the wonder of life. Become aware of your "guest status" in this brief moment in time and space. Be thankful. Exude gratitude. It heals.

## An Important Thing You Can Do

It's time for another page in your Wellness and Recovery Journal. Complete the following sentence:

I am so happy and grateful now that _____.

Express your gratitude—every hour of every day.

# #49

## PRACTICE
## UNCONDITIONAL
## LOVING

Loving heals. Even though there may be times when we are lost in the abyss of our physical maladies or buried in the agony of our emotional awfulizing, with each moment comes a new opportunity to choose loving. This is a decision that truly heals.

I prefer the word *loving* over *love*. It denotes the action necessary to bring the idea of love to life. Love is not loving until it is released, until it is intentionally given.

Loving without conditions is an intentional choice we make to determine what is coming *through* us rather than what is coming *to* us. The choice to love means we don't have to wait for the medical test results, the doctor's assurances, the elusive remission, or the hoped-for cure. We can choose to love now, this moment. And the next moment. And the next. We always have this power of choice, regardless of the circumstances. This choice heals.

Consider this perspective. The crippling fears surrounding cancer are actually the absence of love. The fear is like darkness that is merely the absence of light. You don't solve a problem of darkness by yelling at it or trying to strike at it. If you want to get rid of the darkness, you turn on a light.

So it is with fear. You don't fight it. You replace fear with love.

This is a profound and radical call, not some live-with-loving-feelings suggestion. Loving is more than a thin veneer. Loving is an act of heroism and courage of the highest order. You should not seek or even expect accolades. Unconditional loving is not a decision surrounded by pomp and circumstance. Most often is has to do with small choices. "How do I choose to respond to this person?" "How might I focus on the positive?" "How can I best help another person?" "How can I best love myself?"

By most standards, the conditions and circumstances of cancer do not inspire loving. Taken by themselves, the conditions may elicit despair; the cancer journey has many such moments. But we can take the loving action anyway! Invariably, the result is a renewed sense of hope that results in a strong biochemical "live" signal to body, mind, and spirit.

Loving starts with self-loving. You can hope to know wellness only from a position of personal emotional and spiritual strength. Self-loving is the wellspring of this vital force. Affirm your great value; cancer does not detract from your self-worth. Self-loving is the root of recovery for thousands of patients.

Does loving seem too difficult a task? Does your mind say that you can never be at peace until the cancer is gone? Do you feel that a total and complete physical cure is the only acceptable answer? Does it seem impossible to love with the sword of cancer balancing precariously over your head?

Love anyway. Focus on the love that comes *through* you and direct it to others. For if you love, you will be well.

Loving is the first and last word in healing, the great balm that quiets distress, the only real "magic bullet" against cancer, and the strongest vaccine to combat malignancy.

Our greatest enemy is not disease but despair. Unconditional loving is the healer.

## An Important Thing You Can Do

It is decision time. Decide to practice unconditional loving for the next hour. And the next hour, and the next. You will know healing—something far greater than a cure.

# #50

---

# SHARE
# THIS
# HOPE

Now that you've invested time reading this book and following at least some of the steps, you're aware that there is much you can do to improve your well-being. Your choices and actions really do make an enormous difference. In partnership with your medical team, you are on the pathway to healing.

But most people don't know these powerful truths. Or if they do, they have only a vague acquaintance with the strategies, not a working knowledge. They deserve more.

Share this hope with others who have been diagnosed with cancer. Discuss these ideas. Encourage one another. Make it your new priority to walk the path of wellness with someone else. This has the cumulative effect of helping yourself while helping another.

I invite you to contact us. We have a free e-newsletter for you, plus a variety of helpful wellness resources. Believe it: you have a caring partner in your journey.

**Cancer Recovery Foundation International**
**www.cancerrecovery.org**

# EPILOGUE:
# YOU
# HAVE
# A FUTURE

This is not the end of a book. It is the beginning of a lifetime journey.

While cancer is certainly a serious illness, anyone who has fought the battle knows that it is as much a psychological and spiritual battle as a physical one. They also know what a meaningful contribution the mind and spirit can make.

I encourage you to begin the journey this hour. No matter how much time you think you may have to live, make the decision to live today—fully! Make the profound choices to forgive and to love. This leads to a better life and, as thousands of us believe, a longer life as well.

Let this illness be your new beginning. Choose to be well this moment. A hopeful, happy future can be yours. Choose it now. It's truly the essential thing to do when the doctor says, "It's cancer."

# APPENDIX A:
# IF CHEMOTHERAPY
# IS RECOMMENDED

Throughout this book you may have sensed that I am cautious, even skeptical, about chemotherapy. If so, you are correct. I want you to know of my belief, some have called it a bias, in order to balance it with your own research and convictions regarding your treatment choices.

The guiding dictum of the Hippocratic oath is, "First do no harm." Chemotherapy does not measure up to this standard. Simply put, the goal of chemotherapy is to harm cancer cells by poisoning them in order to disrupt their ability to grow and multiply. Sometimes, in some cases of cancer, it works.

However, in this process your host defense system is typically compromised and, at high doses, often irreparably damaged. Further, tumors that initially respond to treatment frequently develop a resistance to these toxic drugs. And while a tumor may respond a second time, the response is often at a much lower level of effectiveness.

Worse, with long-term use, the body is typically weakened to a point where less-invasive alternatives have little chance to effectively rebuild immune function, extend life, or yield quality-of-life gains.

That said, let me also state that chemotherapy does have its place. Good science shows chemotherapy to be efficacious in producing long-term remission in most cases of Hodgkin's disease, acute lymphocytic leukemia, and testicular cancer. Chemotherapy is also shown to be effective in a handful of relatively rare, mainly childhood cancers including Burkitt's lymphoma, lymphosarcoma, and choriocarcinoma. Used with surgery and/or radiation therapy, chemotherapy plays a role in the successful treatment of Wilms' tumor, Ewing's sarcoma, rhabdomyosarcoma, and retinoblastoma.

In addition, research shows chemotherapy to be effective in extending life by several months in many cases of ovarian cancer and small-cell lung cancer. However, chemotherapy by itself does not seem to affect a cure. Further, quality of life typically suffers.

Sadly, "adjunctive" (additional) chemotherapy has become the standard of care for breast cancer. I call this "sad" because the evidence is simply not conclusive. At best, there may be a very small statistical advantage, at most a 2–4 percent point gain, in survival rates for those who receive chemotherapy. But this small gain must be weighed against the very real potential for collateral damage caused by the same treatment. The single most common long-term problem is impairment of the heart function. In other words, while chemotherapy may seem to marginally increase survival rates, it substantially increases the risk of other potentially serious health problems.

For postmenopausal women with breast cancer, a statistically stronger case can be made for the hormone blocker raloxifene, now the preferred choice over tamoxifin. However, both these drugs have been linked to other health problems, including blood clots, stroke, and increases in endometrial cancer, uterine cancer, and liver cancer. These hormone blockers are perhaps best suited to a narrow group of high-risk premenopausal breast cancer patients. The goal there is to reduce the risk of cancer spreading to the second breast. Evidence suggests the hormone blockers help.

Chemotherapy's one other area of limited success is colon cancer. There is still no conclusive evidence of its effectiveness except after lymph node involvement. Sadly, once again, even though the clinical evidence is mixed, the current Western practice says to treat with chemotherapy in virtually all cases of colon cancer.

After studying this carefully for over a decade, I believe oncologists in the Western tradition are administering chemotherapy to more patients, across a wider spectrum of malignant disease, based on the hunch that it may show results. The cancer community has tended to extrapolate their narrow successes and consider nearly all patients, especially those with metastatic or recurrent cancer, as candidates for chemotherapy. All this to the exclusion of high-level nutrition, exercise, mind-body, and faith-health regimens.

In short, those are my concerns about chemotherapy and its overuse. I consider this an urgent warning to patients everywhere. I ask you to understand clearly, through your own independent research, what chemotherapy can be expected to do and what it cannot be expected to accomplish. Then, make your own decision.

Science says, "Show me the data." The data says, beyond the cancers mentioned above, there is no proof of chemotherapy's effectiveness in the form of large-scale randomized clinical trials. The truth is the widespread use of chemotherapy is not based on convincing scientific data. Even in those cancers where some outcomes can be observed, current chemotherapy regimens alone very often fail to produce a cure or a longer life, or improve the quality of life. It is the multifaceted integrated cancer care approach emphasized throughout this book that is crucial to understand and implement.

*Special note to patients who choose chemotherapy:*

Having stated my very real reservations, I want to state that chemotherapy may be right for you. One important aspect of any treatment's success is the belief the doctor and the patient bring to the process. It's understandable that many oncologists believe in chemotherapy based on tumor response or "shrinkage." Theoretically, it makes sense. If you can reduce the tumor burden, perhaps the body can rebuild immune function.

From the patient's viewpoint, it is also understandable. Since chemotherapy is widely accepted and supported by the medical community, since insurance will reimburse for its administration, and since billions of cancer research dollars are invested in investigating this treatment modality, it comes with a great deal of upfront cultural support. With all that evidence, it seems believable.

If you do choose this therapy, I urge you to use extreme caution in approving high-dose chemotherapy. There are now dozens of studies on the use of high-dose chemotherapy across a broad spectrum of cancers. The results are almost universally disappointing. There are simply very few studies that show better outcomes with high-dose chemotherapy compared to those receiving a lower dose. This data directly challenges earlier studies and widely held assumptions regarding increased survival rates with higher doses.

Is there a middle ground? Fractionated-dose chemotherapy, smaller doses infused over an extended period of time, may be one. The toxic effects of the drugs are typically minimized because the lower doses do not create systemic toxicity. In fact, there exists an increasing body of evidence from Europe that low-dose chemotherapy appears to stimulate immune function. Although most conventionally trained Western oncologists dismiss this evidence, I predict this homeopathic "less-is-more" approach will become widely accepted.

Finally, if you choose to undergo chemotherapy or have already had chemotherapy, study carefully the following chapters: Adopt This Nutritional Strategy During Treatment (section 21) and Determine Your Nutritional Supplement Program (section 22). Start strengthening and rebuilding your immune system immediately.

# APPENDIX B:
# COMPLEMENTARY
# THERAPIES AND
# SELF-HELP TECHNIQUES

Two out of three cancer patients embrace one or more complementary or alternative practices. The information that follows is an overview of the major options. Your goal should be to obtain more complete information of the subjects that are of interest to you. Then you can design an appropriate integrated-care program of your own.

**Question:** When the subject is nontraditional cancer treatments, what should you expect from your oncologist?
**Answer:** Indifference.

For the most part, twenty-first-century oncology has limited time for, or interest in, complementary and alternative therapies. The biomedical model is tightly focused on surgery, radiation, chemotherapy, and hormonal therapy. Do not expect enthusiastic endorsements of approaches outside these core orthodox treatments.

If you were to expect anything beyond indifference, expect

criticism. The conventional cancer community's "party line" on diet, nutritional supplements, and other more natural treatment approaches remains decidedly negative. Only the rare oncologist will bridge the world between mainstream and complementary medicine, support you in the process of taking charge of your situation, and work step-by-step with you toward the recovery of your health.

Know this: a patient's interest in nontraditional cancer treatments is seen as a personal affront by most Western oncologists. It's as if the patient is saying, "Your ideas are not enough." Truth is: they are not. Do not expect to receive positive support for your complementary and alternative efforts from a conventionally trained and practicing oncologist.

You can typically expect more advice and support on complementary and self-help techniques from an informed nursing staff. The control of treatment side effects is the most common nurse-provided information. Their coaching might be expected to include both pharmaceutical options as well as more natural approaches. Look for referrals to community-based organizations for visualization, massage, relaxation, breathing techniques, comfort, and support.

Let's briefly review the most common components of integrated cancer care:

## COUNSELING

Counseling within a holistic model is considered a central component of the healing process. Support through talking, through genuine give-and-take communication, is critical. It will help you become aware of your needs, define your questions, and determine how to go about receiving answers. In a real sense, this increased awareness is the heart of the entire holistic approach.

Millions carry a bias against counseling, thinking it is simply about relief of emotional distress. But transpersonal counseling, assisting to help the individual explore his or her needs from a whole-person perspective, is much more. Cancer challenges everything—from our physical body to our thoughts, feelings, significant relationships, and spirituality, as well as the environment in which we live.

While the initial focus of such counseling may be to help cope with the diagnosis and treatment of an individual's cancer, the counseling quickly becomes more expansive and even a cocreative experience. Discovery of the true self is both enlightening and supportive, encouraging the individual to access all resources—physical, emotional, and spiritual.

Perhaps the key issue of a transpersonal counseling approach is spiritual. It can help us identify what our soul and spirit are yearning for. Not surprisingly, a good number of cancer patients find ambiguity—on the surface they are engaged in actively fighting illness but at a deeper level they are blocked by a seemingly unsolvable problem that leads to despair or even the need to let go and die. Connecting with our deepest reality through transpersonal counseling often establishes great truth, peace and, ultimately, a healing of a higher order.

## GROUP SUPPORT

Cancer Recovery Foundation's earliest work was focused exclusively on establishing psychospiritual support groups. The distinct advantage of this focus over a medical/clinical information approach is helping cancer patients discover the many abilities they possess and then implement them to overcome their present challenges. By focusing on what is possible, the aim is to give the individual a clear picture of the most effective way forward. Doing so within the context of mutual support among people in similar situations is extremely helpful.

The aim of group support is not to expose an individual's feelings. However, the process of group interaction can make it easier and safer for many people to express emotions, even safer than with family, friends, or a one-to-one counseling session. The group is also extremely effective in working together to identify common beliefs and patterns that may be obstructing progress towards self-acceptance and well-being.

## CREATIVE THERAPIES

Art and music can bring freedom, giving people permission to express what they find difficult to put into words. These techniques require no previous training or even talent and ability. Often they are linked with group support. The central benefit is to release the more playful, joyful, and creative aspects of our individual natures. There is healing in the energy and fun we took for granted in our youth.

## Art Therapy

Art therapy reconnects people with their own creativity. Work done in art therapy can help people discover a sense of empowerment and control in the often disempowering and out-of-control cancer experience. Art therapy can also be cathartic, releasing insights into recovery.

Creating with water colors, acrylics, oils, charcoal, pens, markers, clay, paper, glue, or whatever they choose often suspends people in the moment, allowing them to become absorbed and involved. This is exceedingly beneficial in its own right because the mind can be at ease from its typical worries.

All art therapy is deemed to have high artistic merit. The symbols are important. It's joy and peace that the patient-artist is after. Positive expectations can be strengthened, emotional conflicts can be resolved, and a deepening awareness of one's spiritual dimension can be revealed—all through art therapy.

## Music Therapy

Music has a long historical link with healing. The idea of music as a healing influence that could affect health and behavior is as least as old as the writings of Aristotle and Plato. Today a substantial body of research supports the efficacy of music therapy.

There are some common misconceptions about music therapy. That the patient has to have some particular music ability to benefit from music therapy—he or she does not. That there is one particular style of music that is more therapeutic than all the rest—this is not the case. All styles of music can be useful in effecting change in a patient's life. The individual's preferences, circumstances, and need for treatment, and the patient's goals help to determine the types of music he or she may use.

Be it actively playing music or simply listening to music, it has been demonstrated that music therapy can help people control anxiety, express feelings, lift spirits to a higher level, and even relieve pain. The positive shifts can result in a physiological boost.

## Spiritual Healing

Spiritual healing, and for our purposes this will include laying on of hands, is perhaps the very oldest of the healing arts. This practice is part of the beliefs and practices of many religions. Based in the belief that we are all children of God, the practice seeks to reconnect the individual to the source that heals.

Increased connection with God certainly helps with coping. It can also dramatically improve one's understanding and acceptance of life circumstances. For many individuals, this reconnection further provides a strong reason for living, even a mission for one's life.

Spiritual healing can be brought about by prayer being offered by a healer or healers, by personal prayer, or by self-healing exercises. Spiritual healing rests in the belief that an individual's spirit, this universal life force that animates each of us, often becomes depleted. Through prayerful focused intention, the healer is able to tune in to that loving energy and bring it to whomever needs it, including themselves. The result is a restoration in the balance of body, mind, and spirit.

For the past two decades, I have studied with some of the most-respected and best-known healers. These various practitioners each have their own beliefs and practices. Results vary. However, there is this important insight: spiritual healing has its most powerful results when patients have their own strong personal beliefs and connect with a healer who shares those beliefs.

Lasting spiritual healing takes place in the quiet of one's spirit. For the most part, it will not be found in the arenas, on the stages, or under the television lights. There may be a celebration of healing in that environment, but the actual healing is found elsewhere.

I have repeatedly observed one important dynamic of spiritual healing. The turning point is to be found where the individual seeking healing expresses a sincere desire for, and an invitation asking for, God to live in and through him or her. That invitation is very often followed by an inner turning toward a transcendent peace, a profound change toward a life characterized by a more loving and spiritual perspective. What follows is a lifting of the spirit, a joy, and a new healed life.

## Energy Work

### Acupuncture

Acupuncture originated in China millennia ago. The therapist uses very fine needles that are inserted into the body along "energy channels" within the body. Primarily known as a tool to manage pain, it can be useful as an adjunct to pain medication. It is also known to lessen side effects of conventional treatment; it's effective in decreasing nausea and fatigue. Patients report improved sleep, digestion, and appetite.

## Shiatsu

Shiatsu is a form of acupressure that originated in Japan. It combines healing touch with a noninvasive acupuncture in order to help rebalance energy. It reduces stiffness, pain, fatigue, and stress, and it improves energy and sleep.

## Therapeutic Touch/Reiki

Therapeutic touch or Reiki decreases stress and anxiety, helps reduce fatigue, aids in recovery from physical/emotional trauma, and helps minimize side effects of conventional cancer treatments.

### BODYWORK

## Alexander Technique

Decreases muscle strain, nerve pain, chronic pain, fatigue, and postsurgical weakness.

## Chiropractic

Useful for musculoskeletal pain, particularly for the lower back. Decreases joint and muscle aches and releases tension. Improves range of motion. Increasing claims for improvements in general health and well-being.

## Craniosacral

Head and neck massage. Treats muscle tension, injury, structural misalignment, and nerve dysfunction. Decreases stress.

## Massage

Primarily used in pain management. Provides emotional and physical relief. Relaxes nervous system and decreases anxiety. Helps sooth tension, and improves circulation, breathing, posture, and range of motion.

## Polarity Therapy

Emotional and physical energy balancing. Improves circulation. Relieves pain and stiffness. Increases energy, flexibility, and clarity.

## Rolfing®

Deep muscle bodywork. Decreases stress, chronic pain, and stiffness. Improves breathing, mobility, energy, and posture.

## MIND-BODY THERAPY

### Biofeedback

Mind/body focus. Decreases cancer treatment side effects, insomnia, pain, depression, and tension. Studies show improved immune response. Excellent research to document positive effects.

### Guided Imagery

Similar to biofeedback. Reduces side effects, pain, and stress. Aids in emotional coping with cancer. Assists in preparing for anticipated situations such as surgery or chemotherapy. Helpful in decision-making. Improves mental health and control. Reduces need for pain medication. Research shows increase in natural killer cell activity as a result. Guided imagery is perhaps the most important of the complementary techniques for cancer patients.

### Meditative Practices

Includes meditation, yoga, qigong, and tai chi. These practices improve relaxation and reduce stress, anxiety, and depression. As a result, immune function is supported along with improvements in heart and respiration function. Like guided imagery, these practices are among the most documented complementary approaches.

## ALTERNATIVE MEDICAL PRACTICES

### Ayurveda

Supports and promotes good health through a nutritional program. Also used to manage side effects of treatment and stress management. Herbal treatments and colonics are often part of this program.

### Homeopathy

European in origin, homeopathy administers prescriptive symptom-like medications, usually in low potencies. This triggers the body's own ability to combat illness and disease. Today, homeopathy is increasingly associated with fractionated-dose chemotherapy, where the physician monitors the results of a dilute-potency treatment before prescribing anything further. Minimizes side effects.

### Naturopathy

This is an umbrella term to describe the original basis of natural, holistic, and alternative medicine. Its fundamental belief is that nature heals and that the body is inherently self-healing. Naturopathy gives appropriate support to therapies such as diet, herbs, nutritional supplements, exercise, heat, massage, bodywork, counseling, and relaxation therapy. Improves immune functions and strengthens physical response.

### Osteopathy

Osteopathic medicine helps improve structure and function of the musculoskeletal system. Particularly effective for chronic pain, mobility, and postsurgical healing. Also emphasizes nutritional support.

# APPENDIX C:
# NATURAL NONTOXIC
# ALTERNATIVE CANCER
# THERAPIES

One of the reasons for my commitment to expand Cancer Recovery Foundation globally is to educate people to the fact that a wide variety of excellent anticancer therapies do exist, albeit not yet in Western medicine. This book is limited to helping people put in place an integrated cancer care program. Typically, that includes conventional medical care such as surgery, radiotherapy, chemotherapy, and/or hormone therapy.

Other treatments simply cannot be covered within the scope of this book. Yet they need exposure, too, especially for people who have had disappointment after disappointment with conventional medical options. What follows is a partial list of the alternative treatments that I know, firsthand, have effectively helped people with cancer extend life and improve quality of life. I offer this list without evaluation or endorsement. A simple Google search will yield information for your consideration.

| | |
|---|---|
| Antineoplaston therapy | Chaparral |
| Hydrazine sulfate | Dr. Moerman's Anti-cancer diet |

| | |
|---|---|
| Hoxsey therapy | DMSO/hematoxylon therapy |
| Pau d'arco | Essiac |
| Wheatgrass therapy | Revici therapy |
| Chelation therapy | Mistletoe (Iscador) |
| Traditional Chinese medicine | Macrobiotics |
| Gaston Naessen's 714-X | Oxygen therapies |
| Immunoaugmentive therapy | Hyperthermia |
| Gerson therapy | Enderlein therapy |

Three stand out as holding exceptional promise for wide-scale use. Antineoplastons seem especially promising for brain tumors. Iscador, widely used with much success in Germany, is plant-based and actually derived from mistletoe. Plus hyperthermia, or heat therapy. It is time, past time, that these three treatments are routinely integrated into conventional oncology care globally.

My aim here is to communicate to you a simple awareness that many other treatments exist. Many of these are superior to the conventional cancer treatments offered in North America and much of the world where Western medical practices are prominent.

If like me, you are diagnosed with stage IV disease, make it your number one priority to explore these alternatives. Choose the one that engenders your confidence.

# My Cancer Recovery
# Contract

*I hereby devote the next year of my life to "Creating Wellness."*
*In addition to my chosen treatment, I commit my full intent*
*and focused efforts to getting well again.*

## I will:

### Medical:
- Continually research and understand all my treatment options;
- Implement a treatment plan that has my highest confidence; and
- Monitor the results both personally and with my healthcare team.

### Nutrition:
- Consume a plant-based whole food diet;
- Eliminate refined "whites;" add bountiful fresh "colors;" and
- Implement a vitamin/mineral/herbal supplement program.

### Exercise:
- Discover a physical activity that is "fun;"
- Commit to daily "fun;" and
- As a result, capture the emotion of joy.

### Attitude:
- Become an expert on the mind/body connection;
- Focus my mind on healing, not on the problems of treatment; and
- Constantly affirm my health improvement.

**MEDICAL**
**NUTRITION  EXERCISE**
**ATTITUDE  SUPPORT**
**SPIRITUAL**

### Support:
- Nurture relationships that uplift;
- Put toxic relationships "on hold;" and
- Bond with others who are deeply committed to survivorship.

### Spiritual:
- Live in constant connection with God.
- Release, let go and forgive all hostility in my life;
- Embrace gratitude as my way of life; and
- Practice unconditional love in thought, word and deed.

*I hereby commit to traveling this incredible path to living well. And I affirm,*
## "I am cancer-free, a picture of health! Thank you, God!"

_____     _____
Signature            Date

*Please sign, date and place this contract where you will see it every day. For ongoing support, please contact www.CancerRecovery.org*

Copyright © 2008 Cancer Recovery Foundation International